DO YOU
REALLY
NEED THAT
PILL?

DO YOU
REALLY
NEED THAT
PILL?

HOW TO AVOID SIDE EFFECTS, INTERACTIONS, AND OTHER DANGERS OF OVERMEDICATION

JENNIFER JACOBS, MD, MPH

Foreword by David L. Katz, MD, MPH, FACPM, FACP, FACLM

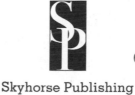

Skyhorse Publishing

Skyhorse Publishing books may be purchased in bulk at special discounts for sales promotion, corporate gifts, fund-raising, or educational purposes. Special editions can also be created to specifications. For details, contact the Special Sales Department, Skyhorse Publishing, 307 West 36th Street, 11th Floor, New York, NY 10018 or info@skyhorsepublishing.com.

Skyhorse® and Skyhorse Publishing® are registered trademarks of Skyhorse Publishing, Inc.®, a Delaware corporation.

Visit our website at www.skyhorsepublishing.com.

10 9 8 7 6 5 4 3 2 1

Library of Congress Cataloging-in-Publication Data is available on file.

Cover design by Rain Saukas

Print ISBN: 978-1-5107-1564-6
Ebook ISBN: 978-1-5107-1565-3

Printed in the United States of America

The information provided in this book is the result of extensive research into the medical literature. It is intended only as a reference for those who want to learn more about the risks and benefits of medications for many common disorders. The decision as to whether or not to take a drug should be made, as always, by each individual in collaboration with his or her medical provider.

For Jacob, who was born and grew along with this book.

Table of Contents

Foreword

I suspect all of us have some (and most of us have abundant) reason to appreciate the remarkable prowess of modern medicine. I routinely ask members of my audiences to raise their hands if a loved one has been touched by heart disease, cancer, stroke, or diabetes—just several of the most prevalent chronic diseases and leading proximal causes of premature death in industrialized societies around the world. By the time I complete that short list, every person in every auditorium with very rare exceptions has a hand in the air.

Those hands, representing people we love, are all the reason most of us need to respect ongoing advances in biomedical science. We are beneficiaries of new drugs and new technologies that can, and do, save lives. Heart attacks can now be aborted as they occur, rather than observed with passive dismay as they were only decades ago. The same is sometimes true of strokes; they, too, can be aborted before doing permanent damage. Type 2 diabetes is treated ever more effectively with ever safer drugs. Cancer mortality rates are declining steadily with advances in chemotherapy.

My family is certainly among the innumerable beneficiaries of modern medical technology and pharmacotherapy; as am I, personally. When I contracted anaplasmosis (a potentially lethal tick-borne illness), I was very grateful for the infusion of antibiotics that produced a full and fairly prompt recovery. When I tore my ACL (and sometime later, my other ACL . . .), I was grateful for the skill of my orthopedic surgeon, the technological advances that led to arthroscopy (joint surgery performed with a fiber-optic viewing device), and the modern anesthesia that let me sleep blissfully until it was all over. (Waking up to the pain afterward was not much fun!)

And finally, as an internist who has cared for patients for most of the past twenty-five years, I have made routine use of diverse medications and know for sure in many cases—and hope in many others—to have done much good and provided genuinely needed help as a result.

But Jennifer Jacobs is quite right that overuse of medication in our culture is a serious problem. She is quite right that the benefits of medication may be the tip of a proverbial iceberg, made highly visible and positioned in the most favorable light through the efforts of Big Pharma and their Madison Avenue representatives. The bulk of the story may well lie below the waterline. In this book, Dr. Jacobs shines a light where it is most needed, where the shadows tend to be densest. She is quite right to ask you to ask: do you *really* need that pill? As our nation struggles to confront an opioid addiction epidemic that is among the great crises of modern public health, this book could scarcely be more timely.

I have long shared this concern with Dr. Jacobs. As a specialist in lifestyle medicine, disease prevention, and health promotion, I am among those concerned with the divide between the "health" care system of which we speak, and the "disease" care system we actually have. We tend to wait for disease we know how to prevent routinely with healthy lifestyle practices to develop, and then treat it with drugs. The situation is one step more ominous than that: our culture generates corporate profits by marketing willfully addictive junk food that makes people sick, and then more corporate profits by marketing the drugs to treat the rampant chronic disease we didn't need to get in the first place.

By and large, we have a disease care system, and since all systems have a vested interest in propagating and perpetuating themselves, this one has a vested and pernicious interest in prevalent disease. There is no shortage of actual disease, alas, but the system takes no chances. At times, as Dr. Jacobs notes, disease is invented to justify the use of a drug. At times, what was once a variant of normal behavior is redefined as pathology.

I have grappled personally with that last one. My one son is the youngest of my five children. While all of his sisters were very active kids, my son—now eighteen—was hyperkinetic at a whole different level. My wife and I were well aware that his rambunctiousness—and that's really what it was—was apt to earn him a diagnosis of ADHD, and a Ritalin prescription. We wanted none of that. My son inspired one of my signature rants: the proper remedy for rambunctiousness in a child is recess, not Ritalin! Since I work in public health, we were able to do more than rant, and actually developed, and studied, a program of brief, intermittent activity bursts for application in schools, called A-B-C (Activity Bursts in the Classroom) for Fitness. We made the program freely available, and it's now in hundreds if not thousands of schools throughout the United States and the world. And by the way, my son is a perfectly healthy young man, headed off to college—and no, he never took Ritalin.

As Dr. Jacobs describes in detail, the problem is poignant in children, but more prevalent and often even more urgent in older adults. Most disease care is concentrated in our later years, and much of the prevailing pharmacotherapy is concentrated there as well. Combine a culture prone to overmedicalize, with genuinely prevalent chronic disease, plus a system in which specialists may tend to treat a condition or body part rather than the whole person, and you have a perfect formula for polypharmacy-induced mayhem.

This book provides expert guidance on navigating past just that peril.

There are, at times, kinder, gentler, safer, and very effective alternatives to medications. At times, there are not. There is a sentiment in the modern world that "natural" is synonymous with safe, but that is misguided. Rattlesnake venom and botulinum toxin are natural. So, too, the smallpox virus, and the polio virus. The vaccines that have eradicated smallpox and nearly eradicated polio are, of course, science; as is the germ theory that enabled us to understand the underlying cause and effect in the first place.

Do you *really* need that pill? The answer may be yes, or no. What you certainly *do* need is expert guidance and balanced judgment to answer this critical question reliably. Find them here.

David L. Katz, MD, MPH, FACPM, FACP, FACLM, earned his BA degree from Dartmouth College; his MD from the Albert Einstein College of Medicine; and his MPH from the Yale University School of Public Health. He is the founding director of Yale University's Yale-Griffin Prevention Research Center, immediate past president of the American College of Lifestyle Medicine, and founder/president of the True Health Initiative.

Introduction

As a family physician, I have become increasingly alarmed at the number of medications that people take, especially ones that are not really needed. And with my training in public health, I am concerned that this troubling epidemic of overmedication is not being recognized or reported by the health-care community. It is an epidemic that hits older adults especially hard, but people of all ages and from all walks of life are often victims of this increasingly common problem. Some drugs are essential—like insulin for people with diabetes, antibiotics for various infections, and drugs for high blood pressure and other heart problems, to name a few. However, many others are optional, unnecessary, or have side effects that are more dangerous than the condition they are treating.

I came face-to-face with this problem when my husband and I spent ten days taking care of his eighty-eight-year-old mother after she was discharged from the hospital. Two weeks earlier, she had gone to the emergency department with severe diarrhea. As is typical in busy EDs these days, the doctors did no diagnostic tests to find out why she had diarrhea. Instead, she was treated by a standardized protocol that postpones testing unless the problem doesn't go away.

Her problem—a severe fecal impaction—did not go away. Rock-hard stool was lodged in her colon, which paradoxically caused diarrhea, as her body tried to move waste material past the blockage. If the ED physician had done an adequate medical history, he would have found out that Arlyn had been taking large doses of morphine—an opioid drug notorious for causing constipation—as well as stool softeners and laxatives for many months.

He would have noticed that she was taking *Lasix*, a powerful diuretic that causes loss of fluids from the body and can lead to dehydration. But instead of receiving a thorough investigation of her illness, she was sent home with a routine antibiotic prescription.

The diarrhea continued until a grandson stopped by one morning and found her incoherent and confused. He took her back to the hospital where she was found to be severely dehydrated and in acute kidney failure. She was hospitalized and treated with intravenous fluids. Her condition improved after a few days, after which she was sent home.

Arlyn's discharge diagnosis from the hospital was *polypharmacy*, a term I had not heard before. But by looking at the list of prescriptions from her last visit to her primary care doctor, I could see there was a big problem. She was on *thirteen* different drugs, including three for high blood pressure, three painkillers (including two different strengths of morphine), an antidepressant, two laxatives, and a potassium supplement to counteract the effects of the blood pressure medicine.

In addition, she had been given two inhalers for chronic lung disease and was told to take low-dose aspirin to prevent blood clots and nitroglycerin for chest pain. Why the morphine? As I later learned, this strong, addictive opiate was often prescribed to elderly patients. It is relatively inexpensive and provides excellent pain relief. However, it is metabolized in the kidneys, causing problems in older patients who have reduced kidney function.

After reading through the list, I was shaken. Polypharmacy indeed! It was a wonder that she was still alive. If I, thirty years her junior, took all of these medications every day, I do not think I could function. In the first place, no one really understands how all of these drugs interact with one another. And it would take a computerized spreadsheet to keep up with the schedule of pills— *three times daily, three tabs at bedtime, every morning, twice daily after meals, every four to six hours, as directed.* How could she cope? No wonder she ended up in the hospital with kidney failure. It's amazing she didn't have a nervous breakdown as well.

HOW COMMON IS OVERMEDICATION?

Arlyn's experience stimulated me to investigate the problem of overmedication. Taking multiple drugs is not necessarily overmedication. But the more drugs you take, the more likely you are to be taking ones that you don't need or ones that are causing you more harm than good. I was shocked to learn that 40 percent of people over age sixty-five regularly take five or more prescription drugs, a number that has tripled in the past twenty years. Sixty-five percent take at least three, while as many as 12 percent take ten or more daily drugs. A study of recently hospitalized patients aged sixty-five or older reported that 23 percent of them were taking sixteen or more drugs as they left the hospital. This is particularly troubling in the light of research showing that one in five prescriptions for people in this age group is inappropriate.

While more common in seniors, the use of multiple medications is prevalent throughout the entire US population. In one survey, 21.8 percent of adults took three or more prescription drugs in the previous month. The use of five or more drugs nearly doubled in the time period between 1999–2000 and 2011–2012, from an estimated 8.2 percent to 15 percent. Fifteen percent of the total adult population involves millions and millions of people—clearly the risk of overmedication is growing. Even in children, prescription drug use is relatively common—the same survey reported that one in four children had taken at least one in the previous month.

THE DANGERS OF OVERMEDICATION

Taking multiple medications increases your risk of side effects, drug-drug interactions, medication errors, and accidental overdoses. All of these can lead to serious medical injuries and even deaths, as well as significant costs to the health-care system.

In 2017, the US Food and Drug Administration reported that almost four hundred and fifty people in the United States die each day from the side effects of drugs. Can you imagine the headlines and panic if four hundred and fifty people died each day in terrorist attacks or airplane crashes? Yet we hear very little about this in the media. A national survey found that those who took five or more drugs have nearly twice the risk of having a side effect, and that there are more than four million outpatient visits each year for side effects, or adverse drug reactions (ADRs). The more drugs you take, the more likely this is to occur.

In addition to adverse reactions, the National Academy of Medicine estimates that 1.5 million people in the United States are harmed each year from drug-related errors. In US hospitals alone, the cost of these errors has been estimated to result in $3.5 billion in extra costs to the health-care system. Another problem is unintended drug overdoses, which first exceeded traffic accidents as the leading cause of accidental death in the United States in 2008, with an estimated 15,000 deaths from pain medications that year. In 2014, there were more than 47,000 deaths from accidental drug overdoses and by 2016, the number of drug overdose deaths reached 64,000.

These problems are not confined to prescription drugs—people also can take unnecessary over-the-counter drugs, vitamins, minerals, and herbal supplements. All of these increase the risk of overmedication. Misuse of nonsteroidal anti-inflammatory drugs (NSAIDs), such as aspirin and ibuprofen, leads to more than 100,000 hospitalizations and 16,000 deaths per year. Taking multiple drugs also increases the risk of other medical problems. The risk of falling is twice as likely in those taking four or more drugs, while people over age sixty-five taking ten or more drugs are *eight times* more likely to suffer a hip fracture than those taking one or no drugs.

THE CAUSES OF OVERMEDICATION

Overmedication is a direct reflection of the growing sales of prescription drugs over the past decade, which totaled $380 billion in the United States in 2016 and is projected to reach $590 billion by 2020. Mayo Clinic researchers reported that over the course of one year, 21 percent of the population received a prescription from five or more drug groups, 17 percent took an antimicrobial agent, 13 percent took an antidepressant, 12 percent were prescribed at least one course of a narcotic painkiller, and 11 percent took a cholesterol-lowering drug. More than a quarter of all women ages fifty to sixty-five were taking an antidepressant, a shocking statistic. Specialists who don't talk to each other, television ads by pharmaceutical companies, and increasing demands on doctors' time are but a few of the reasons for the rise in drug prescriptions. More than $14 million per *day* were spent in 2015 for drug advertisements aimed directly at consumers. This tells me that something is wrong—as a fellow family doctor once told me, "If they have to advertise a drug to patients, it's not really needed."

Another cause of overmedication is the use of one drug to counteract the side effects of another. This creates a vicious cycle of prescribing a medication and then treating the side effects with a new drug, and then another for new side effects, until the patient and the health-care provider cannot remember where the cycle began. Or, a side effect of a drug is mistaken for a new diagnosis and then a second (or third) drug is prescribed.

UNDERSTANDING THE PROBLEM

The problem of overmedication continues to grow. Almost everyone has a story about a friend, coworker, or loved one who has suffered from unnecessary or excessive drugs. In this book, you will hear some of these stories, as I strive to answer the following questions:

- What are the dangers of taking too many drugs?
- Why are we having this epidemic of overmedication?
- Which drugs do you really need and which ones are doing you more harm than good?
- How do you broach the subject with your doctor about taking too many drugs?
- What are some alternatives to taking conventional drugs?

In Part One, I will talk about the dangers of overmedication, such as drug-drug interactions, adverse side effects, medication errors, and unnecessary prescriptions, as well as side effects masquerading as a new illness that requires more medications. I will also explore the causes of overmedication, including "made-up illnesses"— those invented by pharmaceutical companies to sell more drugs. In Part Two, I will cover the benefits and harms of common drugs for many chronic health problems, including high blood pressure, diabetes, high cholesterol, osteoporosis, acid reflux, depression, and chronic pain.

Finally, in Part Three I will show you how to talk to your health-care providers about the medications you're taking and how to decrease them, when possible, through positive lifestyle changes and alternative healing methods.

It is my hope that after finishing this book, you will share your insights with others, beginning the conversation that is necessary to end this deadly epidemic. I am convinced that just as now we look back with horror at the use of leeches and bleeding two centuries ago, our descendants will regard our current overreliance on pharmaceutical drugs with equal dismay.

Part One

Defining the Problem

Chapter 1

The Dangers of Taking Too Many Pills

There are a host of dangers from taking too many medications—adverse side effects, drug-drug interactions, unnecessary and inappropriate drugs, mistakes, and accidental overdoses. It is important for you to be aware of these dangers, since your health-care provider may be too busy to thoroughly evaluate your medications.

ADVERSE SIDE EFFECTS

Most drugs have minor side effects, such as dry mouth, nausea, and headache—nuisances but not serious enough to stop taking something that you need. What many people don't realize, however, is the magnitude of serious and life-threatening adverse effects of many common drugs.

I was shocked almost twenty years ago when I first heard about the study that reported that 106,000 people in the United States died annually in hospitals from side effects, or adverse drug reactions (ADRs). This made side effects of medication the fourth leading cause of death, after cancer, heart disease, and stroke. Even more disturbing, these deaths occurred in cases where the medications were *taken as directed*. That's right—they were not drug errors or overdoses. They were deaths from medicines that were given and taken correctly, according to the recommended guidelines. This study, which stunned the medical community, also reported that there were 2.2 million dangerous adverse reactions every year in hospitals. Again, all of them were cases in which the medications were prescribed in recommended doses.

Things have not improved in the ensuing years. According to the US Food and Drug Administration (FDA), the number of reported deaths from ADRs reached more than 164,000 in 2017, a number that has more than tripled since 2006. Think about it for a minute. One hundred and sixty-four thousand deaths per year divided by 365 days means about *450 deaths each day* from adverse drug reactions.

The FDA also reported that there were more than 900,000 serious ADRs in 2017—nearly 2500 each day—including hospitalizations and life-threatening or disabling reactions. The number of ADRs reported by the pharmaceutical industry tripled between 2006 and 2014 to more than 1.2 million per year. These statistics are likely the tip of the iceberg, since according to the Institute for Safe Medical Practices, the pharmaceutical companies submit incomplete reports in more than half of cases. These companies also delay the reporting of many serious events, including deaths, as reported in a 2015 medical journal.

Not only has the incidence of adverse drug reactions increased with the growth of overmedication, but the risk of an ADR is much greater in those who take multiple drugs. Researchers from Harvard Medical School reported that the number of outpatient visits for adverse drug reactions in the United States nearly doubled from 2.7 million in 1995 to 5 million in 2005. Patients taking five or more different medications were twice as likely to suffer an ADR than those taking only one or two. The authors also reported that more than 100,000 hospital admissions each year were due to ADRs.

I first began to question whether drugs might cause more harm than good when Susan, a young woman in her late twenties, came to see me as a patient during my family practice residency many years ago. She complained of mild pain in her finger joints after spending the afternoon working in her garden. Following the accepted practices of the time, I prescribed an anti-inflammatory drug, *Naprosyn*.

The next time I saw Susan, the joint pain had disappeared, but she now complained of frequent stomachaches and fatigue. Her stomach was very tender when I touched it. Laboratory tests revealed that she was anemic and had blood in her stool. I realized that all of this was due to the side effects of her medication, which had caused bleeding of her stomach lining. I told her to stop the *Naprosyn* and prescribed an iron supplement for the anemia. She then became constipated from the iron. Susan finally decided that she could live with occasional joint pain and stopped taking all of the drugs.

Newly Approved Drugs

Taking newly approved drugs can be risky, since dangerous side effects are not always recognized right away.

Vera, a perky sixty-five-year-old real estate agent with osteoarthritis in one knee, came to see me several years ago for a routine exam. She told me that her knee pain was gone and that she was feeling twenty years younger after starting on a new drug, *Vioxx*, at the recommendation of her internist.

When I checked her blood pressure, however, it was dangerously high. I didn't understand this, since she was taking the same dosage of medication that had kept it under control for many years. Since the *Vioxx* was the only change in what she was taking, I advised her to discontinue it. Her blood pressure came down immediately and stabilized with no further problems.

Other patients were not so lucky. *Vioxx,* a nonsteroidal anti-inflammatory drug (NSAID), was prescribed to more than 80 million people worldwide for five years before its toxicity was recognized and it was taken off the market. During that time, 88,000 to 138,000 Americans had heart attacks from taking *Vioxx* and 30 to 40 percent of them had died, according to an FDA official.

In general, I do not recommend that my patients take a newly approved drug until it has a safety record of several years. Research studies are usually carried out on a small number of relatively healthy adults before a drug is approved by the FDA. They often do not show the long-term side effects, especially in older people or in those who have other health problems. And drug companies do not always report side effects in a timely manner. As was the case with *Vioxx,* it can take the combined experience of millions of users before evidence of the drug's toxicity becomes evident.

The FDA has an early warning system to help its doctors identify safety problems with newly approved drugs. It is based on the FDA Adverse Event Reporting System (FAERS), which collects reports of ADRs from drug manufacturers, physicians, pharmacists, and the general public to look for patterns of side effects from specific drugs. In 2015, the FDA fell so far behind in publishing these "watch lists" that it took a harsh report from another government agency, the Government Accountability Office (GAO), to motivate it to catch up. In the meantime, doctors and patients were not told about warnings of possible adverse events, including indications of an increased stroke risk from a new class of diabetes drugs, SGLT2 inhibitors.

Anticholinergic Drugs

Many common drugs—antidepressants, painkillers, and antihistamines, to name a few—are anticholinergic. These drugs inhibit acetylcholine—a chemical in the brain that helps transmit information from one brain cell to another—and have been linked to an increased risk of declining mental function, dementia, and even death. Half of all people over age sixty-five are taking at least one anticholinergic drug. Studies have shown that the ill effects are cumulative—the more of these drugs you take, the greater the chance of mental impairment.

In a ten-year study of more than 3,000 people aged sixty-five and older, those taking the highest cumulative doses of anticholinergics were found to have one and a half times the incidence of dementia and Alzheimer's disease compared to nonusers. Magnetic resonance imaging (MRI) has shown increased shrinking (atrophy) of several areas of the brain in those taking these drugs. This was correlated with memory problems and other types of intellectual dysfunction. Taking only one anticholinergic drug for just two months can decrease mental functioning by 50 percent, while people taking three or more for at least three months have three times the risk of mental impairment. It is possible that the increasing number of people with dementia and Alzheimer's disease is related to the use of these drugs. Common anticholinergic drugs include:

- Antihistamines—*Actifed, Antivert, Atarax, Benadryl, Dimetapp, Dramamine*
- Antidepressants—*Norpramin, Paxil, Sinequan, Tofranil*
- Antipsychotic drugs—*Thorazine*
- Urinary incontinence drugs—*Detrol, Ditropan, Enablex, Urispas*

- Antispasmodic drugs—*Bentyl, Librax,* scopolamine patch
- Antinausea drugs—*Compazine, Phenergan*

A complete list of anticholinergic drugs can be found at: http://www.agingbraincare.org/uploads/products/ACB_scale_-_legal_size.pdf

Side Effects from Nonpharmacologic Drugs

Adverse effects also occur from nonpharmacologic drugs. Data collected over a ten-year period estimated that approximately 23,000 visits to emergency departments and 2,000 hospitalizations each year were due to adverse reactions to dietary supplements. While these numbers are considerably lower than the five million annual visits reported for pharmaceutical drugs, it is important to be aware that these products are not without risk.

Side Effects Masquerading as a New Illness

Another risk of taking multiple medications is what is sometimes called a *prescribing cascade.* This occurs when the side effects of a drug are mistaken for symptoms of a new illness and a new drug is prescribed. Subsequent side effects of the new drug are then treated with yet another drug, creating a vicious cycle of more and more medications.

My ninety-four-year-old uncle was the victim of a prescribing cascade. My cousin Samantha called me one day, alarmed that her dad had gone downhill precipitously and could barely function. He had become severely confused, incontinent, and was now having symptoms his doctor said could be Parkinson's disease.

She told me that when Uncle Eph had visited his internist for a routine checkup two months previously, the doctor had asked him to count backward from one hundred by sevens and then administered a word memory test. From these results, he concluded that my uncle was suffering from the early stages of Alzheimer's disease. This struck me as odd, since thought my uncle was unusually sharp for his age when I had spoken to him by phone. The doctor prescribed a new drug, *Aricept*, which he said would slow down the progression of the disease.

Shortly afterward, Uncle Eph started having trouble holding his urine. He was given a medication for incontinence, *Ditropan*—an anticholinergic. Over the next few weeks, he became increasingly confused and forgetful as well as somewhat belligerent. Thinking that these symptoms were due to rapidly advancing Alzheimer's disease, his internist then prescribed an antipsychotic drug. After that, my uncle started to have trouble walking and began making involuntary repetitive hand motions. When the internist suggested that this new problem might be Parkinson's disease and prescribed something else, my cousin called me in a panic.

This was shortly after my experience with Arlyn taking too many drugs, so I reviewed Uncle Eph's history and looked up the side effects of the medications he was taking. I found that the drug *Aricept* can cause incontinence and that *Ditropan* is associated with memory loss and confusion. Finally, I already knew that antipsychotic drugs can cause symptoms that mimic those of Parkinson's disease.

I told Samantha to stop giving her dad all of these drugs and to wait two weeks. Sure enough, in a couple of weeks Uncle Eph was back to normal. He could hold his urine, was no longer confused, and had resumed his daily walks around the neighborhood. Perhaps he still was imperfect in subtracting sevens from one hundred, but that seemed a small price to pay for his improved health.

I found the whole episode to be incredibly ironic: the drug *Ditropan*, which my uncle took for a side effect of *Aricept*, caused him to have the very problems—memory loss and confusion—that the first drug, *Aricept*, was supposed to prevent. Luckily my uncle had a medical person in the family who could research his condition and sort out the problem. I wondered, though, about all the victims of this multiple medication disaster who don't have an informed friend or family member to advise them.

HOW TO AVOID ADVERSE SIDE EFFECTS

- Read the package inserts of your medications and look them up on the Internet to find out the common side effects you might experience.
- Ask your pharmacist if there are any specific side effects to watch out for, and tell your doctor if you experience any of them.
- Be aware of the potential side effects of over-the-counter drugs (OTC) and supplements you are taking.
- Minimize or eliminate your use of anticholinergic drugs.
- Avoid taking medications that are newly approved.
- Be alert for any new symptoms that you have experienced since starting a drug, and tell your health-care provider about them.

DRUG-DRUG INTERACTIONS

Another problem to consider with overmedication is the risk of drug-drug interactions. The more different medications you take, the higher the probability you will have a drug-drug interaction. If you take two different medications each day, the potential for drug interactions is approximately 6 percent. The risk rises to 50 percent with five drugs per day and is as high as 100 percent with eight. Approximately 15 percent of older adults sixty-two to eighty-five years old were at risk for a drug-drug interaction in 2011, according to published research. This is nearly double the estimated 8.4 percent at risk reported for 2006. Many drug interactions involve nonprescription medications—OTC drugs, dietary supplements, and herbal products. During the same five years, the number of people over age sixty-two taking five or more medications, including nonprescription ones, increased from 53.4 percent to 67.1 percent.

Pharmacists are trained to alert people when there might be a dangerous interaction between the drugs they are taking, but this only can happen when someone regularly uses the same pharmacy. Seeing several health-care providers also contributes to the problem, since the cardiologist you see for heart problems might not know about the drugs your rheumatologist has prescribed for arthritis or vice versa. While there is considerable knowledge about the interaction of one drug with another, not much is known about the combination of three or four or more drugs taken together.

Warfarin

Some drugs carry more of a risk of interactions with other medications. The blood thinner warfarin (brand name *Coumadin*) is one of these. It is commonly given to prevent blood clots in people with heart irregularities, like atrial fibrillation, and to people who have recently had surgery. It has a very narrow range of safety since too much of it will cause brain hemorrhages and other types of excessive bleeding. Several drugs, including the anticholesterol drug simvastatin (*Zocor*), painkillers like aspirin and ibuprofen, and OTC garlic pills, vitamin E, and ginseng, greatly increase the risk of bleeding when taken with warfarin.

There is evidence that the use of warfarin along with the diabetes drugs glipizide (*Glucotrol*) or glimepiride (*Amaryl*) dramatically elevates the risk for severe hypoglycemia (low blood sugar) in older adults. In a study of emergency department (ED) visits, this combination of drugs was associated not only with hypoglycemia, but also with fall-related bone fractures and altered consciousness.

Serotonin Syndrome

Serotonin syndrome is a potentially life-threatening condition. It occurs from the interaction of two or more drugs that cause the body to produce or inhibit the breakdown of serotonin, a chemical manufactured by nerve cells.

Symptoms of serotonin syndrome include restlessness or agitation, nausea and vomiting, rapid heartbeat, diarrhea, loss of coordination, increased body temperature, and hallucinations. In the case of eighteen-year-old Libby Zion, who was admitted to a New York hospital in 1984 with a high fever and uncontrollable jerking, the combination of the painkiller *Demerol* with an antidepressant she recently had started taking led to her death from cardiac arrest within seven hours. Although more than 7,000 people develop serotonin syndrome each year, surveys have shown that 85 percent of physicians have never heard of it, nor do they know the drugs that can cause it. Some of the medications that can cause serotonin syndrome are:

- Antidepressants—*Celexa, Cymbalta, Effexor, Paxil, Prozac,* and *Zoloft*
- Antimigraine medicines—*Amerge, Axert, Depakene, Imitrex,* and *Tegretol*
- Pain medications—opiates, fentanyl (*Duragesic*), and meperidine (*Demerol*)
- OTC cough syrups containing dextromethorphan (*Robitussin DM*)
- Herbal products—ginseng and St. John's wort
- Illicit drugs—amphetamines, cocaine, Ecstasy, LSD, and opiates
- Antibiotics—ciprofloxacin (*Cipro*) and fluconazole (*Diflucan*)

Other Common Drug Interactions

Other common interactions to watch out for are:

- Lisinopril (for blood pressure) with potassium supplements—dangerously elevated blood potassium level that can lead to heart attacks or even death
- Proton pump inhibitors (PPIs) (for acid reflux) or niacin (a B vitamin) with anticholesterol statin drugs—increased risk of muscle damage
- Antihistamines with blood pressure medicines— increased blood pressure and heart rate
- Ginkgo biloba with thiazide diuretics (for blood pressure)—increased blood pressure
- St. John's wort with warfarin and many common drugs for asthma, depression, erectile dysfunction (ED), heart failure, and high cholesterol—decreases blood levels of the medicines

Arlyn's Drug Interactions

By the time my mother-in-law was released from the hospital, her morphine had been reduced by half. But Arlyn had begun to suffer the symptoms of narcotic withdrawal—agitation, sleeplessness, and depression. The discharging doctor had prescribed a tranquilizer and an antidepressant to deal with these symptoms. The interaction of these two medications—both anticholinergics—caused Arlyn to become disoriented and severely confused. When my husband, Dean, and I arrived at her apartment the following morning, we found that she had tried to make hot chocolate during the night by putting an aluminum packet of Swiss Miss into the microwave and turning it on. The charred remains were all that were left.

After her weeklong stay in the hospital, she was still constipated. We encouraged her to eat fruits and vegetables and walk up and down the hall outside her apartment. She was unsteady on her feet and complained of dizziness. When Dean took her blood pressure, it was dangerously low. He called her family physician, who told us to taper off two of her blood pressure medications and the antianxiety pills, a combination that can lower blood pressure too far.

Alarmed at the adverse effects of the medications Arlyn was taking, we decided to see if there were any other drug-drug interactions. I found a website, www.drugs.com, that lets you enter all the drugs someone is taking and then gives an analysis of possible drug interactions.

After I entered the list of Arlyn's medications, the website reported potential dangers from *one major* drug interaction, *nine moderate* drug interactions, and *two minor* ones. The most serious potential problem was stomach bleeding that could occur as a result of the interaction between the emphysema drug *Atrovent* and potassium chloride, which she took for the side effects of the diuretic *Lasix*.

The morphine that she took had potential interactions with *five* of her other drugs. Two of them, the drug gabapentin (*Neurontin*) for nerve pain and the antidepressant desipramine (*Norpramin*), carried a warning that said that, in combination with morphine and/or each other, they could cause dangerous respiratory and nervous system depression, especially in "elderly or debilitated patients." Since Arlyn had chronic obstructive pulmonary disease (COPD), depression of the respiratory system especially concerned us.

The three drugs she was taking for blood pressure, amlodipine (*Norvasc*), prazosin (*Minipress*), and furosemide (*Lasix*), were dangerous to take along with morphine due to the possibility of hypotension, or low blood pressure. On the other hand, the low-dose aspirin, which she was taking as a preventative for heart attack or stroke, could decrease the effects of her hypertension medicines, leading to abnormally high blood pressure and stroke. We hoped that cutting out two of the hypertension drugs would prevent both of these potential problems.

Finally, we found a possible interaction that may have contributed directly to Arlyn's kidney failure—the combination of the laxative (senna) with the diuretic (*Lasix*). Taking these two together, especially in the long term as Arlyn had done, depletes the body of fluids and essential salts, leading to dizziness, fatigue, dry mouth, muscle cramps, and ultimately kidney failure.

HOW TO AVOID DRUG-DRUG INTERACTIONS

- Be aware that the more drugs you take, the more likely you are to have a serious, even life-threatening interaction.

- Check your drugs on websites like www.drugs .com to see whether there are any potential drug interactions.
- Give your health providers a list of all of the medications you are currently taking and ask them to review this periodically.
- Be aware of any signs or symptoms you might have that indicate a drug interaction and talk to your health provider about your concerns.
- Know that antidepressants, antihistamines, and warfarin most often have interactions with other drugs.
- Discontinuing a drug or switching to a different one could save your life, but check with your doctor first.

MEDICATION ERRORS

Everyone makes mistakes, including patients, doctors, nurses, and pharmacists. And the more drugs that you are prescribed, the more likely it is for someone to make a mistake. Drug errors occur in all health-care settings—hospitals, nursing homes, assisted living facilities, doctor's offices, and even at home.

A study published more than fifteen years ago reported that 7,000 Americans died each year from medication errors, accounting for one out of every 131 outpatient deaths and one out of every 854 hospital deaths. Another study found that 1.5 million people are harmed each year by medication errors, resulting in $3.5 billion in extra medical costs to the US health-care system.

I could not find any more recent statistics about drug errors. But we do know that the average number of prescriptions written for people over age sixty-five nearly doubled between the years 2000 and 2010—from 28.5 per person to 49 per person. We can only guess that as the number of drugs people take has increased, the number of deaths and injuries from drug errors has also grown.

The most common drugs that cause medical errors include insulin products, anticoagulants (blood thinners), antibiotics, and narcotic pain relievers (opiates). In hospitals, many of these errors occur from shift changes in staff, fatigue, distractions, and excessive workloads.

Outside of hospitals, data analyzed from poison control centers in the United States found that *one medication error occurs every eight minutes* in young children. One-quarter of these happened in children under age one. Half of the drug errors in children involved pain medications and cold and cough preparations. Confusion over directions for liquid dosages, which are sometimes written as teaspoons and other times as milliliters, has led the American Academy of Pediatrics to call for metric units to be used in all pediatric dosing.

Mistakes When the Medicine Is Prescribed

More than half of all drug errors occur when medicines are prescribed, such as:

- the doctor ordering the wrong drug or dose
- prescribing a medication for which there was a known interaction with another drug the patient is already taking

- failing to note a drug allergy
- not telling the patient enough about the medicine

Sometimes, especially in EDs and hospitals, medication is given to the *wrong patient*. This can happen as nurses are making their rounds of multiple patients or when doctors prescribe medicines for several patients at one sitting.

Poor handwriting, the use of abbreviations, and putting decimal points in the wrong places can also lead to medication errors. A common abbreviation used on a prescription is QID, which means four times a day. But this can be confused for QD (every day) or QOD (every other day), depending on the handwriting. A dose for .5 milligrams can be misread as 5 milligrams, or 5.0 milligrams might be read as 50 milligrams. An error that changes the dosage by a magnitude of ten can be extremely dangerous.

People thought that the use of electronic health records would help prevent prescribing errors but that is not always the case. Doctors now use drop-down menus, which can create errors when the mouse is clicked in haste above or below the desired drug or dosage selection. Doctors can be confused about which patient they are prescribing for when handling multiple patient charts at one time. Primary care physicians spend an average of sixty-six minutes a day responding to electronic health record notifications, making it more likely for them to skip over ones that might caution about a possible drug error.

Mistakes also are commonly made in monitoring the use of medications, such as inadequate laboratory testing of blood levels of a drug or a delayed response to symptoms of drug toxicity. Patients with impaired liver or kidney function metabolize drugs more slowly than other people and should have their blood levels checked frequently.

Mistakes When the Prescription Is Filled

Some drug errors are caused by confusion between similar drug names, again due to poor handwriting by doctors. Examples of confused names are *Inderal*, a cardiac drug, and *Adderall*, an amphetamine used to treat attention deficit hyperactivity disorder (ADHD). Can you imagine the problems that giving an amphetamine to someone with a heart condition could cause? *Paxil*, an antidepressant, is easily confused with *Taxol*, an anticancer drug. Up to 25 percent of all drug errors reported to the US government are due to confusion in drug names.

Colin, a twenty-two-month-old toddler, had a horrible cold. His nose was constantly running and he was sneezing and coughing so much that he couldn't sleep. His doctor prescribed *Zyrtec*, an antihistamine, to dry up the secretions from his nose. Colin's dad picked up the liquid pediatric syrup from the pharmacy, but after taking it for twenty-four hours, the boy was no better. His doctor was stumped—he couldn't understand why the *Zyrtec* hadn't helped. Further investigation revealed that Colin had received a bottle of *Zantac,* which is used for stomach problems, not *Zyrtec*. Since both medicines are sold to pharmacies in amber-colored pint bottles, and they were stored alphabetically next to each other on the pharmacy shelf, the pharmacist had pulled out the wrong one. Luckily Colin suffered no ill effects.

Mistakes When the Medicine Is Taken

Mistakes in taking medications cause another one-fifth of preventable drug errors. Patients take doses incorrectly or at the wrong times, forget to take doses, or stop medications too soon. It is easy to understand how this happens, especially with people over age sixty-five, who account for 34 percent of all prescriptions written in the United States. Many are prescribed multiple doses of more than five different drugs daily, each with its own dosage schedule.

At a time in life when memory is waning, adhering to complicated directions about time of day, relationship to food, and frequency of administration is more than many older people can handle. One medicine three times daily, another twice a day, a third four times daily, several at bedtime, and still more "as needed"—it is mind-boggling to imagine keeping up with that daily regimen.

A study of nearly 500 adults ages fifty-five to seventy-four looked at how well people followed dosing instructions. Participants were given a hypothetical seven-drug medication regimen and asked to demonstrate how and when they would take all of the medications in a twenty-four-hour period. Only 15 percent of them took the medicines correctly. Medicines that were labeled *twice daily* and those that said *every 12 hours* were not taken at the same time by 79 percent of the participants, even though these instructions mean the same thing.

The authors of the study pointed out that the more cumbersome and harder to remember a medication schedule becomes, the greater the likelihood that people will misunderstand instructions, skip doses, or abandon their drug regimen altogether. They suggested that a standardized four times a day dosage schedule be used to consolidate all of the drugs a person is taking.

Mistakes in taking medications also occur outside the home, perhaps even more frequently. In nursing homes and assisted living facilities, where drugs are often administered by non-nurses, drug error rates of up to 42 percent have been reported. The average number of prescriptions per patient in these settings is high, and there is often a shortage of personnel.

Mistakes with Nonprescription Drugs

Medication errors are not confined to prescription drugs. Misuse of NSAIDs, such as ibuprofen *(Motrin, Advil)*, taken by millions of Americans, leads to 103,000 hospitalizations and 16,000 deaths per year. Acetaminophen (*Tylenol*) is extremely toxic if too much is taken and accounts for more than 40 percent of acute liver failure cases in the United States.

Accidental Drug Overdoses

The most deadly types of medication errors are accidental drug overdoses, now reaching epidemic proportions. In 2009, drug overdoses surpassed traffic fatalities as the leading cause of accidental death in the United States, with nearly 38,000 deaths that year—*one every 14 minutes*. By 2014, fatal overdoses reached 47,000, of which 28,647 were caused by narcotic pain relievers alone. And the Centers for Disease Control and Prevention (CDC) reported that in 2016, more than 64,000 Americans died from drug overdoses.

A big part of the problem is the increased number of prescriptions that are written, especially for opioids, such as morphine, and antianxiety drugs. In 2013, 71 percent of the accidental prescription overdoses involved opioid pain medications while another 31 percent were due to antianxiety drugs. Often those who died were found to have a combination of these two types of medications in their blood.

The rate of opioid overdoses has more than tripled since 2000. During that time, doctors became more lenient about prescribing these narcotic drugs for chronic pain, thinking it was unethical to allow a patient to suffer needlessly. Fortunately, this is finally changing. Acetaminophen with codeine is the most commonly prescribed generic drug in the United

States, far surpassing generic prescriptions for heart-related and other medications. The anxiety drug *Xanax* (alprazolam) is often prescribed for minor anxiety. All of these drugs are highly addictive. When taken in combination with each other or with alcohol, their effects are magnified. The US Centers for Disease Control and Prevention (CDC) has recently released a strong warning to doctors not to prescribe opioid pain relievers and benzodiazipines—used to treat anxiety, insomnia, and seizures—together.

Accidental drug overdoses can happen to people of all ages and lifestyles—they do not occur only in drug addicts. Elderly folks, like Dean's mother, can become dependent on these medications and lose track of how many they have taken. Middle-aged people who are taking them for back pain or after surgery can develop tolerance, needing to take more and more of the drugs to get the same relief. Or someone can unintentionally drink too much alcohol while taking them, a dangerous combination.

Young people sometimes find drugs in the family medicine cabinet and take them for fun. Eighteen percent of twelfth graders reported abusing prescription drugs, such as *Adderall, OxyContin, Ritalin, Valium, Vicodin,* and *Xanax,* in 2016. There have been reports of teenagers ending up in the emergency department after attending a party where various drugs are thrown into a bowl and taken together. Many people have the misconception that since these drugs are approved by the FDA and sold by prescription, they are safe.

Mixing narcotics with antianxiety drugs is risky, since both can depress the central nervous system. Even some OTC drugs, such as antihistamines and sleeping aids, can be deadly when mixed with prescription pain relievers. The actor Heath Ledger is only one of several celebrities who have died from combining too many of these drugs.

My friend Arlene, a former runner and competitive skier, was recovering from knee replacement surgery when she had a run-in with opioid pain relievers. Her knee was healing nicely after ten days, and she was having no pain. Indeed, she felt little of anything—her appetite had diminished to almost nothing, and she couldn't concentrate well enough to read a simple paragraph in a book. When she started having hallucinations, her husband decided enough was enough and took her to the ED. She had lost seventeen pounds since the surgery.

Luckily, the ED physician listened to Arlene's husband and agreed that the combination of 40 milligrams of morphine, which she was taking twice daily for pain, along with the sedative she was given for sleep and the benzodiazepine tranquilizer to help her relax, was just too much for her 140-pound body to handle. She tapered off the drugs and was back to normal within a few days.

Accidental drug overdoses are a natural consequence of our society's reliance on taking drugs—especially too many drugs. When children take stimulant drugs to keep them focused at school, it is easy to understand why they might become adults who think it's okay to take a painkiller such as *Vicodin* for a sore back or *Xanax* when nervous before a job interview. Physicians in the United States prescribe ADHD drugs twenty-five times more often than European physicians. It follows that teenagers in the United States have twenty-five times more access to these drugs than their European counterparts.

The take-home message is that the more drugs you take, the more likely there is going to be a mistake—by your doctor in prescribing, by the pharmacist in dispensing, or by you, in taking them.

HOW TO AVOID MEDICATION ERRORS

- Confirm the name of your prescription when you receive it from your health-care provider and make sure that is what you receive from the pharmacy.
- Keep a list of all your medicines in your wallet or purse, and take it with you to your doctors' visits.
- Ask your doctor to write the reason for each medicine on the prescription so that the pharmacist will write it on the label.
- Make sure you understand the directions on the label about when and how to take each medication.
- Avoid or limit the use of opioid pain medications and antianxiety drugs, especially in combination with each other or with alcohol.

UNNECESSARY AND INAPPROPRIATE DRUGS AND DOSAGES

In 2013, a study reported that the United States spends $200 billion each year—about *8 percent of the nation's health-care expenditures*—on medical care stemming from inappropriate or unnecessary use of prescription drugs. Nearly 60 percent of people over age sixty-five take at least one unnecessary drug, contributing greatly to the problem of overmedication.

The more drugs you take, the more of a risk you have, not only of adverse side effects and drug-drug interactions, but also of impaired mental and physical functioning, broken bones from falls, and even urinary incontinence. Laxatives, anticholesterol drugs, antidepressants, antipsychotics, opiates, high blood pressure drugs, and acid reflux medications are often unnecessary, as we will explore in future chapters.

My concern about unnecessary drugs began early in my career—more than thirty-five years ago while I was a family practice resident at a small Florida community hospital. One night, pleasant sixty-seven-year-old man, who had complained about chest pains earlier in the week, was brought to the emergency department by his son. In order to placate his son, Mr. Lewis agreed to undergo some preliminary tests, even while insisting that he felt fine. When his blood test and EKG results came back, I was surprised to find that he had experienced a mild heart attack within the past few days.

I convinced Mr. Lewis to stay in the hospital overnight for observation. Since he felt well and had no symptoms, I wasn't sure if I should start him on the standard drug protocol for a heart attack. I called my supervising physician, who was at a party and irritated with me for bothering him. He told me to go ahead with the drug regimen. I ordered oxygen, an intravenous beta-blocker, and nitroglycerin for chest pain, and went to bed in the resident's on-call room.

In the middle of the night, I was startled awake by a call from the night nurse, urging me to come right away to Mr. Lewis's room. I found him sitting upright and struggling to breathe. He had developed pulmonary edema—fluid in the lungs—for which I ordered a diuretic to flush out the fluid. When an hour passed with no improvement, I started him on digitalis to stimulate the heart. Nothing helped. As I stood by his bedside, watching his breathing become more and more labored, I felt helpless. I had done everything by the book, yet this nice man, who had been feeling well when I first admitted him, was now fighting for his life.

He lost that fight, taking his last ragged breath early that morning, only ten short hours after arriving at the hospital. The attending physician said that Mr. Lewis probably had a paradoxical reaction to medication, and it wasn't my fault. But I was devastated by the incident and began to question the routine use of the medications I had prescribed for him. If he had stayed home, would he still be alive? Did the drugs I had given him cause his demise?

Unfortunately, the line between appropriate and unnecessary prescribing is sometimes difficult to define. The medicines I prescribed for Mr. Lewis were appropriate, according to the standard treatment protocols, but did the possible good that they might do outweigh their possible harms? This is a question that should be asked whenever any drug is prescribed.

The Beers Criteria

The Beers Criteria is a list of drugs that are considered "potentially inappropriate" for people over age sixty-five. It was first established in 1991 and has been updated periodically, the most recent version published in 2015. The list includes many anticholinergics and drugs associated with serotonin syndrome as well as tranquilizers, muscle relaxants, and heart medications. Two of the twelve medications that Arlyn was taking, an antidepressant and one for urinary incontinence, were on the Beers list.

Tranquilizers on the Beers list—such as *Ativan*, *Valium*, and *Xanax*—have been reported to increase the incidence of Alzheimer's disease by as much as 50 percent in older adults, as well as cause mental impairment, delirium, falls, fractures, and motor vehicle accidents. Yet many people continue to take these medications for anxiety and insomnia. The entire Beers list of potentially inappropriate medications can be accessed at: www.empr.com

/clinical—charts/beers-list-potentially-inappropriate-drugs-for-el
derly/article/125908/.

Drugs That Aggravate an Existing Condition

Some drugs are considered inappropriate because they aggravate
a patient's particular diagnosis, such as an antidepressant that can
cause palpitations in someone who already has a heart arrhythmia
or a pain medicine with a side effect of constipation in someone
who suffers from that problem. Fragmentation within the health-
care system contributes greatly to this problem. Patients visit
different doctors for different health problems, often with little
communication between the various professionals about which
medications they have prescribed.

Sally, an engaging retired history teacher, came to see me for
severe heart palpitations, which I had treated successfully in the
past. She was worried that something terrible was happening. The
palpitations were much stronger than those she had before and
were lasting for several hours at a time.

During the course of our interview, she told me that she had
recently seen an endocrinologist and had been started on thyroxine (a synthetic thyroid hormone) for a low thyroid level in her
blood. When I questioned her, she denied having any symptoms
of a thyroid disorder, such as fatigue, constipation, dry skin, or
weight gain. She said that the endocrinologist had not asked her
about heart palpitations.

Of course, I thought, the thyroxine had aggravated her heart
palpitations. The endocrinologist should have asked about heart
problems before prescribing the thyroid drug. Since Sally wasn't
having any symptoms of low thyroid, I didn't think she needed it.
I advised her to stop taking it and when she returned several weeks
later, the palpitations were gone.

Prescribing Without Adequate Testing

The problem of inappropriate drugs is not confined to older adults. Drugs are often prescribed without doing adequate tests to determine the cause of the problem. As we saw in the case of Arlyn, who was treated with antibiotics for diarrhea when she actually had an intestinal blockage, it has become standard medical practice to treat people with antibiotics without doing an adequate laboratory workup.

Twenty-three million unnecessary antibiotic prescriptions are written each year for viral illnesses such as colds, bronchitis, and sinusitis, despite the fact that doctors know that antibiotics don't work for viral diseases. As a medical colleague once told me, "If I don't prescribe them [antibiotics], patients will just go down the street to another doctor to get some."

This is what happened to Gail, a tax attorney, who was having severe abdominal pains and diarrhea after a diving trip in Mexico. She had been given a prescription for an antibiotic but the symptoms hadn't gone away. Over a period of six weeks she lost twelve pounds and her family began to worry that she had a serious illness. She finally visited a gastroenterologist who found an infection with *Giardia*, a parasite found in contaminated drinking water. The correct antiparasitic medicine cleared up the problem right away.

Treating Minor Health Problems Inappropriately

Inappropriate drug use also occurs when a relatively minor health problem is treated with a strong, potentially dangerous drug. Antidepressant drugs, which have been found to be effective for people with severe, debilitating depression, are a good example of this. They are frequently prescribed inappropriately for patients with mild to moderate depression, even though studies have shown that antidepressants work no better than sugar pills for these people.

The latest estimate is that more than 40 million people receive a prescription for an antidepressant in a given year, including up to 25 percent of middle-aged women. At the same time, there is growing evidence that certain classes of antidepressants are associated with increased violent and even suicidal behavior, especially in teens and young adults.

Millions of people with mild heartburn regularly take proton pump inhibitors, such as *Prilosec and Nexium*, originally approved by the FDA for severe cases and only for fourteen days at a time. The FDA recently issued a warning about an increased risk of hip, wrist, and spine fractures from these drugs if taken for longer than two weeks. And the inappropriate use of antipsychotics, known to cause Parkinson's disease–like side effects, is epidemic, especially among the elderly. A government audit of Medicare claims found that 22 percent of nursing home patients were given antipsychotic drugs unnecessarily.

Palliative Chemotherapy

In what seems to be the cruelest example of inappropriate medication use, there is the now-common practice of using *palliative* chemotherapy for terminally ill cancer patients. This may be appropriate in cases when a person has several months to live. But when there are only days or a few weeks left, this practice can cause unnecessary suffering.

A friend recently told the story of her father-in-law, an elderly gentleman with macular degeneration, a progressive eye disease that distorts and finally destroys vision. He had been diagnosed with pancreatic cancer but was pain-free and quite content. Although she and her husband counseled against it, her sister-in-law convinced their dad to undergo palliative chemotherapy. Within the first week he lost all his vision, quickly followed by the loss of his will to live.

He died shortly thereafter. They later found out that chemotherapy is well known to accelerate the process of macular degeneration.

My own heartbreaking experience with this occurred more than fifteen years ago, with my beloved cousin Loella. A smart and sassy sixty-five-year-old, Loella was the glue that held the extended family together, arranging reunions and always remembering birthdays. She had dodged the bullet, we thought, the previous year when a cancerous mass on her liver was removed and there was no sign that it had spread. But she suddenly became severely fatigued and her doctors found that the cancer had spread to her bones and lungs. By the time I flew across the country and arrived at her bedside, she was semicomatose with a feeding tube snaking down through her nose and an oxygen mask over her nose and mouth.

Loella was in a private room with an adjoining sitting area where much of the family had gathered on the plaid sofa and chairs. I was the only MD in the family and my relatives all looked hopefully to me for an optimistic assessment, which unfortunately I couldn't give. As I stood at her bedside, it was clear to me that it was only a matter of days, if not hours, before she would pass away. I looked at the bags of fluids running into the IV in her arm and noticed one that was not familiar—bright yellow-green and slightly opaque.

When I asked what it was, her son told me it was chemotherapy, which the doctor told him might help her. It was then that I noticed the sores inside her lips and the clumps of hair that were falling on her pillow. I was heartsick. She had told me specifically that she did not want chemotherapy if her cancer returned. She had seen how her husband, Joe, had suffered from it before he died of stomach cancer five years previously. And yet here she was, literally on her deathbed, being tortured by the poison that was dripping into her arm, much too late to be of any use.

We asked them to stop the chemo and Loella died the next day. I don't know what happened in Loella's case, but later learned that hospitals and oncologists make a large profit from chemotherapy; they bill insurance companies and Medicare a hefty increase over the wholesale price that they pay for it.

Cutting down on unnecessary drugs would go a long way in preventing many of the risks associated with overmedication. Many doctors do the best they can for their patients, but they are seriously overworked and constantly bombarded by promotional materials for "new and better" drugs, as we will see in the next chapter.

Inappropriate Doses

You might wonder why there are so many adverse reactions when drugs are taken as directed. One reason: the recommended starting dose for many drugs is too high, especially for the elderly and small adults, including many women. When you take your dog or cat to the veterinarian, the assistant will weigh him in order to determine the correct dosage of a medication. This doesn't happen with people. Prescribing the same dosage for everyone saves time for busy doctors. And one-size-fits-all dosing makes production and marketing of medications cheaper and easier for drug companies, since fewer pill sizes are needed.

Pharmaceutical research is usually carried out on young to middle-aged adults who have only one health problem. Only one drug is tested at a time. As people get older, their physiology changes, slowing the rate at which drugs are broken down and eliminated by the liver and kidneys. Drugs that are safe and effective for younger adults can cause entirely different reactions when taken by the elderly or in combination with other drugs. Yet this often isn't taken into account.

In the book *Overdose: The Case Against the Drug Companies*, author Jay S. Cohen, MD, explores this phenomenon in detail. He reports that pharmaceutical researchers have found that the blood levels of many common drugs rise much higher and last longer even in *healthy* older adults, yet the recommended initial doses by the manufacturers for these products are the same for all adults, regardless of age.

Even in younger adults, dosages are not customarily individualized. A 125-pound woman is usually prescribed the same dose of a blood pressure medicine as a 250-pound man. We know that blood levels of alcohol vary dramatically by body weight, but for some reason this difference is rarely taken into account when drugs are prescribed. An elderly, frail woman in my writing group once told me that she cuts her pills in half to avoid the side effects.

Doses often are not tailored to the individual needs of the patient. This was the case with Sandra, who had come to my office complaining of severe muscle pain and weakness in her legs. A tall, willowy blonde who looked much younger than her fifty-three years, she could no longer run or do aerobics and was finding it increasingly difficult to complete her twelve-hour shifts as an emergency room nurse.

I did a routine physical exam but was unable to find the reason for Sandra's symptoms. Then I reviewed her list of medications. I noticed that she had recently been started on a statin drug, *Lipitor*, to reduce her cholesterol, which was 220. When I was in med school, we were taught that a cholesterol level of up to 240 was normal. Over the years, some say at the urging of the drug manufacturers, the recommended upper end of normal cholesterol level has shifted downward to 200. This has created a huge new market for drugs such as *Lipitor*, which was the number-one-selling drug in the United States when Sandra visited me, with $7.2 *billion* in sales that year. Since then, the generic form of *Lipitor*, atorvastatin, has become available and a different statin, *Crestor*, which did not yet have a generic, was the most commonly prescribed branded drug in the United States in 2014.

Sandra had been prescribed a 10-milligram daily pill of *Lipitor*, the usual starting dose. However, it had brought her cholesterol level down to 150, way below the recommended level. And she was experiencing the same side effects that have been reported by up to *one-fifth* of patients taking statins—muscle pains and weakness. Sandra's initial cholesterol level was not very high and likely could have been controlled by changes in her diet. If she did want to continue taking *Lipitor*, it would make sense to lower her dosage to reduce the side effects.

I looked in my *Physicians' Desk Reference*, the bible of drug prescribing, provided free to doctors by the pharmaceutical industry. I was surprised to find that 10 milligrams was the lowest dose available for *Lipitor*. I also read that at that dosage, the medication causes a 39 percent decrease in cholesterol level, much more of a drop than Sandra needed. After discussing the pros and cons of continuing on the medication, Sandra decided to stop it. Once she did, the muscle pains and weakness disappeared and she was able to bring her cholesterol down to below 200 by diet alone.

I was curious about why the starting dose of *Lipitor* was so high. It turns out that in order for a new drug to be accepted by doctors, it has to be shown to be more effective than what is currently being prescribed. Head-to-head studies are done, comparing the effects of the new drug to one or more of the older ones. An easy way to show that the new drug is better than the old one is to use a higher initial dose.

For *Lipitor*, the standard initial dose is higher than is needed by most people. This leads to increased adverse reactions, especially in those who weigh less and/or are elderly. Although studies have found a direct correlation between the dosage of statins and the number of adverse effects, the lowest dose available of *Lipitor* and its generic version atorvastatin remains 10 milligrams, the same as when it was first introduced more than twenty years ago.

Shortly after I saw Sandra, I learned that the drug company Pfizer had started promoting a *higher* dose of *Lipitor*, 80 milligrams, which cost $35 more per month and was said to be more effective in reducing heart-related deaths. When I reviewed the studies on this higher dosage, I found that although there were fewer deaths from heart disease, there were more deaths from other causes. The total number of overall deaths was the same. There were also five times as many liver abnormalities in those taking the higher dose.

In June 2011, the FDA issued a safety alert about a similar statin drug, simvastatin (*Zocor*), after research showed a 50-fold increase in muscle problems in those taking the 80-milligram dose compared to those on 20 milligrams. The ill effects were strongest in women and the elderly. Since then, higher dose statin drugs have been shown to be no better than lower dose ones in preventing death or complications of heart disease while carrying an increased risk of side effects.

Statins are just one class of drugs which are given in higher doses than often are needed. Blood pressure medicines, arthritis drugs, antidepressants, and many other medications are frequently prescribed in inappropriately high doses, especially in women and elderly folks who have diminished liver and kidney function. And with the increase in overmedication, these adverse reactions are multiplied many times, depending on the number of other drugs a person is taking. It should not be surprising, therefore, that one and a half million people in the United States are hospitalized each year and more than 100,000 die from severe reactions to prescription drugs, taken as directed.

HOW TO AVOID UNNECESSARY AND INAPPROPRIATE MEDICATIONS

- Whenever you are prescribed a new medicine, ask your doctor if it is really necessary.
- If you are over sixty-five, check to see if any of your medications are on the Beers list.
- Do not take antibiotics unless you have a confirmed bacterial infection. Tell any specialists you visit about your other medical conditions and which other drugs you are taking.
- If you are elderly, make sure that your doctor tests your liver and kidney function before prescribing medications.
- If you are small, ask your doctor to prescribe the lowest dose possible of a medication.
- Whatever your size, avoid higher doses of medicines when possible to lessen the risk of side effects.

Chapter 2

Why We Are Taking So Many Pills

A "perfect storm" has given rise to the epidemic of overmedication. Pharmaceutical companies share the biggest part of the blame, encouraging the idea of "a pill for every ill," but doctors and patients also contribute to the problem. Understanding the interplay of factors contributing to overmedication will help you make better choices about your health.

THE ROLE OF BIG PHARMA

It's no secret that pharmaceutical companies make billions of dollars and are among the most profitable companies in the world. And in order to do this, they must sell more and more drugs while downplaying the hazards of taking them. The cost of all prescription medicines in the United States in 2015, including those sold in pharmacies as well as those dispensed in doctors' offices and hospitals, was $457 billion, accounting for nearly 17 percent of all health-care spending. This amounted to $1112 per person in 2014, compared to $782 in Japan, the next highest country in drug spending.

There are many excellent books—listed at the end of this book—devoted to exposing in much greater detail the exploitation and greed of this industry, which puts profit ahead of people's health. But it is important to understand the many ways that drug companies contribute to the problem of overmedication.

Direct-to-Consumer Advertising

Advertising directly to consumers is one way to encourage people to take more pills. The United States and New Zealand are the only countries *in the world* that allow direct-to-consumer advertising. Nearly $5.6 billion, more than *$14 million a day*, was spent in 2015 for drug advertisements, most of these aimed directly at US consumers. These direct-to-consumer ads, which were not allowed by the FDA until 1997, often advise viewers to "ask your doctor" about a particular medication.

The simple truth is that the drugs that are the most heavily advertised to consumers are the ones that are the least often needed. Have you ever seen an advertisement in a magazine suggesting that diabetics ask their doctors for insulin? Or have you watched a doctor on TV tell someone with pneumonia to request a prescription for antibiotics?

The vast majority of direct-to-consumer advertising is on television. The average American TV viewer sees nine drug advertisements each day, adding up to sixteen hours a year, more time than is usually spent with a primary care doctor. And if you watch the evening news shows, you will notice that more than half of the ads are for pharmaceuticals.

Proponents of direct-to-consumer ads say that they educate patients and promote a dialogue with their health-care providers. Opponents say that they misinform the public, overemphasizing a drug's benefits and failing to mention that adopting healthy behaviors might also be a solution to a health problem. These advertisements also downplay side effects, such as those on TV that feature pleasant scenes like a family playing in the park while a voice rapidly reels off the side effects. Or, the adverse effects are shown on the screen in hard-to-read white letters on a yellow background.

Direct-to-consumer ads are also criticized for promoting new drugs before their safety profile is fully known. An example is the pain drug *Vioxx*, which was heavily promoted and had sales reaching $1 billion before it was found to have caused tens of thousands of heart attacks and strokes. These ads also lead to inappropriate prescribing, as when a physician agrees to a patient's request for a drug that is not really needed. One study reported that such requests were made during about 40 percent of doctor visits and were successful more than half the time. The American Medical Association is now calling for a ban on direct-to-consumer advertising of prescription drugs.

Half a billion dollars in 2014 was spent on advertising two of the top five most advertised drugs, *Cialis* and *Viagra*, both of which are marketed for erectile dysfunction. Studies show that only 10 percent of men cannot achieve a full erection and that most requests for these drugs are for occasional problems that are entirely normal.

A member of an FDA advisory panel told a reporter about her experience with a heavily advertised new sleep medication from Merck, *Belsomra*. She said that company records had revealed that "people taking *Belsomra* fell asleep, on average, only six minutes sooner than people taking a placebo and stayed asleep for a mere sixteen minutes longer. Some test subjects experienced worrying side effects, like next-day drowsiness and temporary paralysis upon waking. For a number of people, these problems were so severe that the researchers halted their driving tests, fearing someone would get into an accident." Because of these safety concerns, the FDA ended up approving the drug at a lower starting dosage than the company had requested—a dosage so low that a Merck scientist admitted it was "ineffective."

In the meantime, Merck spent $96 million promoting *Belsomra* in 2015. It was expected to generate $300 million in sales in 2016 and become a bigger blockbuster than the two other leading sleep medications within a decade. This for a drug that is taken in such a low dosage that the company's own scientist said it didn't work. The FDA received more than a thousand complaints about *Belsomra* in the five months between February and July 2015, with nearly half saying that it was ineffective.

Inventing New Illnesses

Not content with treating actual diseases, the pharmaceutical industry has successfully invented new ones, opening up vast new markets to sell more pills. Symptoms that are not at all serious or life-threatening, even those that are only minor inconveniences of life, are being promoted as new diseases with, of course, new medications to go along with them.

I remember the first time I saw a TV advertisement for such a drug. A middle-aged couple was walking hand in hand on a picturesque beach at sunset with sweaters knotted around their shoulders. The distinguished-looking man looked down at his lovely wife and asked, "Do you need to go back now, honey?" "No," she said, smiling, "not yet. I can walk some more." Soft music came to a crescendo as their silhouettes receded into the setting sun. *What the heck are they trying to sell?* I wondered. The answer came shortly—a new drug for the problem of "overactive bladder syndrome"—basically a fancy way of saying frequent urination.

The voice on the advertisement went on to say that "studies have shown a significant decrease in the number of trips to the bathroom" for people taking the drug. Interest piqued, I looked up the research evidence for this new drug, *Ditropan*. Sure enough, in the 5,000 people they studied, there was a statistically significant decrease in the daily number of bathroom trips—from ten to eight. The associated side effects were also significant—constipation, headaches, dizziness, and confusion. *All this for two fewer trips to the bathroom*? I thought.

Ditropan became quite successful, making millions for the manufacturer. In fact, as you might recall, it is the same drug that Uncle Eph took for incontinence, the one that caused him to become highly confused and his doctor to think that he had rapidly advancing Alzheimer's disease. More recently, two prominent European urologists have questioned the concept of "overactive bladder," calling it a vague and ambiguous diagnosis in which very mild symptoms can be classified as abnormal. They also say that this terminology, first coined by the pharmaceutical companies, allows them to market their drugs to a large number of patients, although the results are often not what patients were promised.

Another new illness created by the drug industry is "social anxiety." Sure, there are a small number of people who are pathologically shy and need treatment, but they are rare. According to Shannon Brownlee, in her excellent book *Overtreatment: Why Too Much Medicine Is Making Us Sicker and Poorer*, the public relations firm for the pharmaceutical company GlaxoSmithKline launched an all-out public relations campaign to convince millions of people that they needed this drug. They did this by starting a nonprofit organization, the Social Anxiety Disorder Coalition, which sent out public service announcements alerting people to the symptoms and dangers of this illness. Normal reactions like being nervous before public speaking or feeling awkward and uncomfortable in a new social setting were branded "social anxiety." Sales of SmithKline's *Paxil*, an antidepressant that has been linked to suicidal behavior, skyrocketed to $3 billion in 2002, just three years after it was first approved by the FDA for this condition.

Other new "illnesses" include premenstrual dysphoric disorder, which used to be called PMS, erectile dysfunction, the new name for impotence, and sleep disorder, commonly known as insomnia. In a campaign similar to that of *Paxil* for social anxiety, the establishment of "Sleep Awareness Month" by organizations funded by the pharmaceutical industry has convinced large numbers of people that their occasional insomnia needs treatment. Unfortunately, the side effects of the medicines being sold for these newly defined illnesses are often much worse than the symptoms themselves.

Were there little boys in your elementary school who acted up and couldn't keep their hands to themselves? There is now a diagnosis for these mischievous types—attention deficit hyperactivity disorder (ADHD). In my first-grade class photo, taken in the fifties, Skipper Klein stuck out his tongue while Stanley Levy held up two fingers behind the head of the girl sitting in front of him. Today, they would both be subdued with one or more psychoactive medications such as *Ritalin*, a stimulant to help children focus better in school. While ADHD might be a legitimate diagnosis for some children, in others poor attention is more likely due to factors such as a larger than normal class size, problems at home, an uninspiring teacher, or eating too much of a sugary breakfast cereal.

Most of these optional drugs are advertised heavily on television and in magazines. The most astonishing one, recently shown during the Super Bowl no less, was for OIC—opioid-induced constipation. Have you ever heard of this illness? I certainly hadn't. Not only did it amaze me that there were enough people with this problem to make an expensive Super Bowl commercial worthwhile, but the ad also made it seem commonplace to use opioids, highly addictive narcotic pain drugs that cause tens of thousands of overdose deaths each year.

Rich, a sixty-five-year-old retired Boeing engineer, came to my office one day and confessed, "I just can't get it up at times, Doc." Appearing somewhat embarrassed, he asked if I would give him a prescription for *Viagra*, which he had seen advertised on TV. He told me that his difficulty happened once every month or two, mostly when he was tired from fishing all day or drank more than a couple of glasses of wine. Otherwise, he and his wife had sex once a week or so with no problem.

I reassured him that what he was experiencing was entirely normal and that he didn't need a prescription for *Viagra*. I also explained that the side effects of *Viagra*, which increases the flow of blood to various areas of the body, include heart attacks and that prolonged use can lead to blindness. He thanked me and left the office, visibly relieved. I wondered how many patients with Rich's symptoms were getting unnecessary prescriptions and if the ill effects they suffered outweighed the inconvenience of occasional impotence.

The use of drugs for made-up illnesses is best avoided, no matter how persuasive that guy in a white coat on TV might be.

Influencing the FDA and Congress

Drug companies influence various branches of the government in many ways to increase their sales. The FDA is beholden to pharmaceutical companies because they pay user fees that partially fund the agency. The priority of the FDA is to approve new drugs and do so quickly. This sometimes comes at the expense of safety issues, as with the delay in publishing "watch lists" of possible adverse effects of newly approved drugs.

The FDA cites inadequate staffing and competing priorities as the reason they were not able to keep up with the process of tracking safety issues in 2015, although in the meantime several new drugs received "fast track" approval. As Diana Zuckerman, president of the National Center for Health Research, told *Medscape Medical News*, "In the last year, it has become more obvious that the requirements that FDA has as its first priority are the ones that benefit industry—faster approvals."

The FDA also looks the other way when there are irregularities in research studies of drugs seeking new approvals. An investigative journalism team from New York University found that in many cases when the FDA finds scientific fraud or misconduct, the agency doesn't notify the public, the medical establishment, or even the scientific community. Drugs are then approved by advisory committees that are not informed of these problems.

Why does the FDA do this? When questioned, officials say that they don't want to "confuse the public," among other reasons. But there is also the issue of the "revolving door" between the FDA and the pharmaceutical industry. The commissioner of the FDA appointed in 2016, Dr. Robert Califf, previously led a $200 million research institute at Duke University that received more than 60 percent of its funding from the pharmaceutical industry. Califf also received financial support as a consultant or researcher from more than twenty of these companies. These relationships led many public health advocates and others to question whether he was too close to the industry that he regulated.

Pharmaceutical companies also lobby Congress for a quicker review process of drugs and Congress, in turn, pressures the FDA to speed things up. In 2015, the industry spent nearly $150 million lobbying Congress and federal agencies. Currently, lobbyists are pushing a new law that would allow the FDA to rely less on randomized controlled trials—the gold standard in medical research—in granting drug approvals.

The expansion of Medicare to include coverage of prescription drugs (Part D) was a windfall for the pharmaceutical industry. Not only did it guarantee that the government would pay for millions of people's medications, but it also included a provision that prevents the government from negotiating drug prices. In the United States, the cost of drugs is two to six times higher than in other developed countries. For example, a month's supply of the pain medicine *Celebrex* sells for an average of $51 in Canada compared to $225 in the United States.

Influencing Doctors

There are many ways the drug industry encourages doctors to prescribe more pills. After a busy day of seeing patients, few doctors have the time or inclination to keep up with the dizzying amount of information available about new and existing drugs. They rely on sales representatives, medical journals, professional websites, and continuing education programs, many of which are underwritten by drug manufacturers to provide biased information intended to increase sales of their products.

Payments to Consultants and Medical Schools

According to the nonprofit organization *ProPublica*, the total amount of money paid to doctors and hospitals from drug companies during the period of August 2013 through December 2015 was a staggering $6.25 billion. This included payments for speaking, consulting, meals, travel, and gifts to 810,716 doctors and 1,171 teaching hospitals. This does not include funding for research, nor does it include marketing to physicians by drug representatives.

For example, Pfizer, the world's largest drug manufacturer with total sales of $52 billion in 2016, paid nearly $128 million to 168,928 doctors during the August 2013 to December 2015 time period. To find out if your doctor or hospital received any of these payments, check the website projects.propublica.org /docdollars/.

Even medical schools rely on drug company donations, calling into question the impartiality we would expect in training our new doctors. An article in the *New York Times* told the story of a first-year Harvard medical student who was belittled for asking about the side effects of cholesterol-lowering statin medications after the lecturer had praised their benefits. It turned out that the instructor was a paid consultant to ten different drug companies, including five manufacturers of statins.

Officials at Harvard reported in 2010 that pharmaceutical companies contributed $8.6 million for basic science research and $3 million for continuing education classes on campus in the previous year. They also reported that 149 faculty members had financial ties to the drug company Pfizer and 130 to Merck.

Clinical Guidelines

Clinical guidelines for treating specific diseases are issued by experts, many of whom are paid consultants to pharmaceutical companies. New guidelines that resulted in millions more Americans being prescribed statin drugs for high cholesterol were written by a nine-member panel that included six who had received research grants or consulting fees from at least three of the manufacturers of statin drugs. Similar conflicts of interest have been reported for panels making recommendations for treatment of high blood pressure and obesity.

Pharmaceutical Representatives

There are independent organizations, such as the Cochrane Collaboration and the National Academy of Medicine, that attempt to provide a balanced evaluation of drug efficacy and safety for doctors. But they are up against a virtual army of tens of thousands of pharmaceutical drug representatives who visit busy doctors on their lunch hours, often providing a buffet lunch for the entire office staff. Almost $22 billion of the $24 billion spent on direct physician marketing in 2012 was for these face-to-face sales activities and free samples of drugs.

Armed with the latest company sponsored research, these men and women—frequently attractive former cheerleaders—woo doctors with glowing reports of their company's products. Doctors are invited to expensive dinners and flown to exotic resorts for conferences on the newest advances in treating a particular disease, which usually includes a drug manufactured by the sponsoring company. Pharmaceutical companies also obtain printouts of the prescribing patterns of individual physicians from pharmacies and other sources. They then give this information to their drug representatives, who can target or reward doctors accordingly.

A 2016 study found an association between payments or gifts physicians receive from drug companies and their subsequent prescribing habits. Those who received more payments were more likely to prescribe brand-name drugs, leading to concerns by researchers about higher costs to the health-care system. According to Open Payments, a federal program that collects data about payments made to physicians by drug companies and device makers, 48 percent of all US physicians received payments in 2015. The majority of these payments, which totaled $2.4 billion, were for consulting fees, food, and beverages.

Continuing Medical Education

Doctors are required to complete a certain number of continuing education courses each year in order to keep their medical licenses up-to-date. Many of these classes are underwritten by drug companies to promote their latest drugs and are offered to doctors free of charge. The speakers include faculty members at many top medical institutions who can net tens of thousands of dollars in additional income in consulting fees. Even continuing education programs offered online often are written by doctors that have ties to the pharmaceutical industry.

Company-Sponsored Research

Most doctors rely on medical journals to guide their prescribing practices and assume that the studies published there are accurate and free from bias. Unfortunately, this is not always the case. Pharmaceutical firms fund more than 70 percent of clinical trials, which are research studies done to evaluate how well a new drug does when compared to another drug or a placebo.

It has been well documented that drug-company-funded studies that have positive results are much more likely to be published than those that show a negative or no effect from a drug. In an analysis of seventy-four FDA-registered studies of antidepressants, thirty-seven out of thirty-eight positive studies were published in medical journals while twenty-two of thirty-six negative studies were not published and another eleven of these were published in such a way that conveyed a positive outcome. Studies funded by pharmaceutical companies are also more likely to show a benefit of a drug than those sponsored by nonprofit organizations, such as the National Institutes of Health (NIH). Many medical research articles are "ghostwritten" by in-house employees of pharmaceutical companies. They are then published under the names of prominent physicians who receive research grants, consulting fees, or stipends from the same companies.

The results of published studies are not always accurate. In an analysis of fifty-seven published trials that were identified by the FDA as problematic, researchers found that 39 percent had falsified data, 61 percent had inaccurate record keeping, and 74 percent did not follow the intended study plan. The editor of the highly regarded medical journal *The Lancet* went so far as to suggest that perhaps half of the scientific literature is untrue.

Statistically Significant Results

When doctors read about a study in a medical journal, they most often rely on the abstract a summary of the research findings published at the beginning of each article. They don't have time to read through the details of each and every study, so they focus on whether or not the results are "statistically significant." This is research speak for the odds of how likely it is that there was a real effect from a drug, rather than the results of the study happening by chance. If the odds are less than five out of one hundred (.05) that it happening by chance, then a study is deemed to have statistically significant results. How they determine these odds requires a college-level course in biostatistics to understand.

Skimming through a medical journal and reading only the abstracts, most doctors will accept the findings of statistical significance at face value. But there are many tricks to achieving statistical significance in a study. One way is to have a large number of people participating in a study, such as with the drug for frequent urination, *Ditropan,* that we discussed earlier. If there are thousands of participants, even a small difference in outcomes can be statistically significant.

The recently-approved drug *Addyi*, marketed for "Hypoactive Sexual Desire Disorder (HSDD)" in women, is a case in point. Basically a repurposed antidepressant, studies of *Addyi* were hyped as statistically significant, even though women taking it had on average only one-half additional satisfying sexual encounter each month compared to those taking a placebo. Women taking the drug also had four times as much dizziness and sleepiness and twice as much nausea. At the cost of $800 for a month's supply and with a black box warning to refrain from drinking alcohol, I doubt that many women will be eager for that extra "satisfying" half experience each month.

Another way to improve the chances of statistical significance for a new drug is to compare it with an older one with a weaker strength or an incorrect dosage. *Xarelto*, a new anticoagulant, was compared with warfarin (*Coumadin*), the "gold standard" for preventing strokes and other clotting disorders. In a study of more than 14,000 patients in forty-five countries, subjects in the comparison group were taking the correct dosage of warfarin only 55 percent of the time. It was no surprise that *Xarelto* appeared to be significantly better. The FDA ultimately approved *Xarelto* and it now sells for around $350 for a thirty-day supply, generating sales of $1.5 billion in 2014 alone. This is compared to $4 to $15 for a thirty-day supply of warfarin. Also in 2014, *Xarelto* was suspected of playing a role in over 3,000 serious adverse events, including 379 deaths.

Reports of Adverse Effects

Side effect information reported in studies is often incomplete because, according to one researcher, "Commercial sponsors of these clinical trials may not be motivated to search exhaustively for potential side effects. . . . Many trials do not state clearly how adverse effects were assessed." Data about individual patients from research trials are not always made public for independent scrutiny, despite calls from the editor of the *British Medical Journal* for researchers to do so. Also, research subjects who have a history of certain complaints, such as musculoskeletal problems in studies of statins, are sometimes excluded before the study starts. This effectively eliminates those who might report these side effects in the actual study.

The number of adverse effects reported in medical journals is often much less than the number reported to official regulatory agencies. In a study funded by the German government, only 26 percent of harmful outcomes of studies reported in official documents were reported in medical journals. But unfortunately, doctors rely on medical journals for their information, not official documents, many of which are not even published.

Another factor that undermines the independence of medical journals is that more than 95 percent of the advertising that keeps them afloat comes from pharmaceutical companies. So it is in the journals' best interest to publish studies that are favorable to their advertisers. When one medical journal published a report saying that 44 percent of its drug ads were misleading, companies withdrew their ads and the journal almost folded.

THE ROLE OF DOCTORS

The practice of medicine has become filled with the pressure to see as many patients as possible in the shortest amount of time. Most doctors today are employees of large practices or hospitals and are no longer their own boss. In order to keep up with their quotas, they must rush between exam rooms and limit each visit to five or ten minutes. It is much faster for them to prescribe a drug than to talk about lifestyle changes such as diet and exercise.

The advent of the electronic health record (EHR) has increased the burden of record keeping for physicians, taking time away from meaningful discussions with patients. As we learned in chapter 1, doctors spend an average of sixty-six minutes a day looking at the messages in their electronic inboxes. A recent study of internal medicine residents found that they spent an average of five hours each day entering data into electronic health records, more time than they spent with patients. These factors contribute to long work hours, causing physician burnout and creating problems with their personal relationships at home.

Reimbursement Issues

A new concept called "pay for performance" is being used by insurance companies and hospital networks to reward doctors for following standardized treatment guidelines. For example, doctors are given bonuses for keeping their patients' blood pressure or cholesterol below certain levels determined by expert groups. Never mind that the muscle pain from a statin drug might be more of a problem for an individual than a slightly elevated cholesterol level. Or that driving blood pressure too low in a frail elderly person might make her more likely to fall and break her hip.

It used to be that doctors had time to give advice about healthy living habits. That is no longer the case. A national survey found that doctors counseled their patients about tobacco use and weight reduction in only 14 percent of office visits, about exercise in 17 percent of visits, and about diet and nutrition in 28 percent of visits. This is partly due to reimbursement rates by Medicare, Medicaid, and private insurers, which reward specialists for expensive procedures, such as performing a colonoscopy or inserting a cardiac stent. They do not provide payment to primary care physicians—family doctors and internists—for talking to patients about healthy lifestyles.

This could be changing. A pilot program for people with prediabetes saved Medicare $2,650 for each person who received lifestyle counseling about how to prevent type 2 diabetes. It was recently announced that Medicare would start paying for this type of program nationwide.

Patient Expectations

Doctors also must deal with the expectations of patients. Many people equate going to their doctor with receiving a prescription and feel disappointed if they leave the office without one. Rather than explaining that an antibiotic is unnecessary for a viral infection, such as a cold or the flu, it is less time-consuming for a health provider to just write a prescription. Direct-to-consumer advertising contributes greatly to this problem.

Patients are increasingly seen as consumers of a service that they have purchased and doctors worry about how they are evaluated. Websites that rate a doctor's performance and post-visit surveys by provider networks put pressure on physicians to keep their patients happy. This can mean prescribing drugs that are not needed or scheduling unnecessary procedures.

Fear of Lawsuits

Doctors live in fear of lawsuits. And doing too little is much more of a risk for them than doing too much. As long as they follow established guidelines, doctors don't have to worry about being sued. So to be safe, they often overprescribe. If it is later found that a certain drug is associated with a bad outcome, the manufacturer will be sued, not the physician.

Also, dissatisfied patients are more likely to sue. Being rushed through a medical visit does not allow for the kind of personal relationship between patient and provider that promotes trust and respect. Wisdom and empathy, two qualities that a good physician needs, require spending time with someone, not the five or ten minutes that are allotted for most doctor visits. People who feel like they were treated indifferently or not given a drug they requested might call their lawyer instead of their doctor if a problem arises.

THE ROLE OF PATIENTS

While the majority of the blame for our overreliance on medication falls on the pharmaceutical industry and doctors, patients also bear some responsibility for the problem. If you request a drug you saw in an advertisement, your doctor—who knows the drug is unnecessary—might prescribe it anyway, in order to please you. You may also have the expectation that when you visit a doctor you should get a prescription.

The bigger issue is one that is difficult for all of us to face. It is just easier to take a pill, or two, or five, than to lose weight, cut down on red meat, or get out of bed an hour earlier to exercise. We all lead stressful, hectic lives with multiple responsibilities at work and at home. Taking the extra time to chop vegetables for a home-cooked meal or to lift weights for half an hour requires a commitment to taking charge of your health. Yes, it is easier to take a pill. But as you will see in the coming chapters, lifestyle changes can alleviate many of the health problems for which people routinely take medication. And as you will also see, the long-term side effects of many of these medications are much worse than the problem that is being treated.

WHY ARE WE TAKING SO MANY PILLS?

Because pharmaceutical companies:
- spend $14 million each day advertising directly to consumers.
- invent new "illnesses" that require new drugs.
- pay user fees to the FDA, which also regulates them.
- lobby federal agencies and Congress to the tune of $150 million each year.
- pay nearly $3 billion each year to doctors for consulting, teaching, travel, and meals.
- spend another $24 billion on direct marketing to doctors through drug representatives.
- fund 70 percent of all clinical research studies.
- provide 90–95 percent of the advertising revenue for medical journals.

Because doctors:
- are overworked and pressured to see more and more patients.
- find it takes less time to prescribe a pill than to explain why it is not needed.
- are not reimbursed for discussing lifestyle modifications as alternatives to medications.
- are rewarded for following standardized treatment protocols.
- are concerned about ratings from patients on websites and insurance surveys.
- are fearful of lawsuits.

Because patients:

- request drugs they have seen on TV that they don't really need.
- are disappointed if they visit their doctor and don't receive a prescription.
- find it easier to take a pill than to make lifestyle changes.

Part Two

Seven Medical Conditions and the Drugs You Might Not Need

Chapter 3

High Cholesterol and Cardiovascular Disease

One out of every three deaths in the United States is due to cardiovascular disease (CVD)—which includes heart attacks and strokes. And many people are urged to lower their cholesterol levels to reduce their risk of CVD. But lowering cholesterol is only one of several ways to improve your cardiovascular health. Factors such as smoking, obesity, lack of physical exercise, and poor dietary habits contribute greatly to the development of CVD, as do family history, high blood pressure, and diabetes. Yet most of the emphasis in preventing CVD today is on reducing cholesterol—primarily by taking statin drugs—not on adopting healthy lifestyle practices.

Statins are among the most widely used drugs in the world. In the first quarter of 2016, two of the top seven prescription drugs were statins—atorvastatin, the generic equivalent of *Lipitor,* was number one and simvastatin, the generic of *Zocor,* was number seven. Among brand-name drugs—those that were still under patent protection—*Crestor* (rosuvastatin) was the second-most prescribed in the period of April 2014 through March 2015 with 21.4 million monthly prescriptions generating $5.9 billion in sales. Clearly these are blockbuster drugs.

One-quarter of all Americans aged forty and above are taking statins, including more than half of all men and 40 percent of all women aged sixty-five and older. Overall, an estimated 38.6 million Americans are taking a statin, equal to the populations of Texas and Michigan combined. Some experts believe that nearly everyone over age fifty should take these cholesterol-lowering drugs. But what are the facts behind these popular medicines? Should you take them? And do their possible benefits outweigh the risks of their side effects?

WHAT IS CHOLESTEROL?

Cholesterol is found in every cell of the body and is an essential building block for the production of hormones, vitamin D, and other vital compounds. Three-quarters of the cholesterol in your body is manufactured by the liver and one-quarter enters your body through food. Twenty-five percent of your body's cholesterol is found in the brain, where it is used by cells that transmit information to each other. Without cholesterol you could not think, nor could your body perform many essential functions.

Cholesterol is carried through the bloodstream attached to proteins, forming substances called lipoproteins. The two main types of these are HDL—high density lipoproteins—and LDL—low density lipoproteins. HDL, the so-called "good cholesterol," carries cholesterol from other parts of the body to the liver, where it is eliminated. LDL, or "bad cholesterol," can build up in the bloodstream and contributes to the development of plaque—"hardening"—inside the arteries, leading to heart attacks and strokes.

Is Cholesterol Really a Cause of Heart Disease?

Cholesterol became a culprit in the 1970s after a study of diet and heart disease in seven countries showed a correlation between high cholesterol and coronary heart disease. As a result, people have been advised for the past forty years to reduce the cholesterol in their diets, as well as saturated fats from foods like meat and dairy products. However, a correlation does not necessarily mean that something is a cause.

In a study of more than 500,000 people admitted to the hospital with their first heart attack, 72 percent of them did not have high cholesterol. How can this be? If high cholesterol causes heart attacks, you would think that people having heart attacks would have high cholesterol.

In an analysis of twenty-one studies involving nearly 350,000 people, there was no relationship between the amount of saturated fat in their diets and the subsequent occurrence of heart attacks and strokes. However, this analysis did not include information about other foods these people were eating that might have contributed to heart disease. The American Heart Association released an advisory in June 2017 stating that replacing saturated fats with refined carbohydrates and sugars does not lower the risk of cardiovascular disease. They also reported that replacing saturated fats with polyunsaturated vegetable oils can reduce the risk of heart disease by around 30 percent, similar to that of taking a statin drug.

The Inflammation Theory

For many years there has been suspicion that cholesterol is not the main problem in cardiovascular disease. Some scientists believe that the real cause of atherosclerosis—the buildup of plaque inside the arteries—is a condition known as chronic inflammation. Studies have shown an association between a marker of inflammation in the blood—C-reactive protein (CRP)—and heart attacks and strokes. The theory is that the body produces cholesterol in response to inflammation as a way to protect the arteries. If cholesterol were a *response* to heart disease, not the cause, it could explain the correlation between high cholesterol and heart disease that was observed in the 1970s.

High consumption of refined carbohydrates has been linked to chronic inflammation. As low-fat diets became popular in the past few decades, the food industry added excessive carbohydrates, sugar, and polyunsaturated oils to give foods more flavor. And although the percentage of fat in the average American diet has decreased from 40 to 30 percent during this time, the incidence of obesity has skyrocketed.

A report published in September 2016 revealed that the sugar industry, under the guise of a nonprofit association, paid prominent researchers to write an influential review in the late 1960s and made clear to them that the role of carbohydrates in heart disease should be minimized. This review led to subsequent dietary guidelines focusing on saturated fat as the main risk factor for heart disease and downplayed the role of sugar.

Some doctors think that decreasing saturated fats in our diets has actually increased the risk of cardiovascular disease because it has been replaced by refined carbohydrates and sugars. "It is time to bust the myth of the role of saturated fat in heart disease and wind back the harms of dietary advice that has contributed to obesity," wrote a prominent cardiologist. He went on to say that millions of people are overmedicated with cholesterol-lowering drugs.

PREVENTING HEART DISEASE WITHOUT DRUGS

There is ample evidence that lifestyle modifications can be every bit as effective as taking anticholesterol statin drugs in preventing CVD. Eighty percent of cardiovascular disease could be prevented by changes in three lifestyle factors—diet, smoking, and exercise—according to a study comparing more than 15,000 people in fifty-two countries who had heart attacks to matched controls who had not. Another study of more than 84,000 nurses over fourteen years had similar results, finding that lifestyle modifications could reduce the risk of CVD in women by more than 80 percent.

Karen, a retired real estate broker, knew that her cholesterol had been creeping up for years. When she was sixty-two, she was told by her doctor that her cholesterol was 280—too high—and that she should start taking a statin drug. She told me that she hadn't been wild about the idea of going on statins, since she spent six months every year on a sailboat in Mexico. She was concerned about having a side effect—which she knew could be significant—without having her doctor nearby.

Although she felt that she lived a fairly healthy lifestyle with plenty of exercise and a good diet, she decided to get serious about bringing down her cholesterol level without drugs. After much research, she committed to a one-year program of 1) working out for one hour five days a week; 2) reviewing the foods she ate to cut down on saturated fat, especially the lard found in many Mexican foods; 3) drinking at least 40 ounces of water daily; 4) adding two tablespoons of apple cider vinegar to a cup of hot water daily; and 5) eating oatmeal for breakfast nearly every day.

Karen was holding her breath when her lab results came back a year later, since this would determine whether she would be pressed into taking drugs or not. She was delighted to hear that her cholesterol reading was 202, a 28 percent drop. All the ratios, HDL/LDL, etc., were good. Even her normally reserved doctor gave her a high five and congratulated her on a job well done. The following year, her numbers were still stable. Needless to say, Karen looks and feels great as she continues to sail in Mexico for several months every year. The final reward, she reports, was at her last exam when, after listening to her chest, her doctor said, "Heartbeat of an athlete!"

The Mediterranean Diet and Fiber

Consuming a Mediterranean diet—fish, fruits, vegetables, legumes, olive oil, and whole grains—can reduce heart disease and deaths from all causes by as much as 30 percent, more than the 25 percent reduction that has been attributed to statin drugs. This has been found to be true even in patients who have risk factors such as cigarette smoking, high blood pressure, obesity, or a family history of heart disease.

The protection provided by the Mediterranean diet is likely due to the replacement of saturated fats with plant-based and fish oils, as well as the high amount of fiber found in whole grains, beans, fruits, and vegetables. The more fiber that is eaten, the lower the risk of CVD, according to a combined analysis of twenty-two different studies. For every seven grams of fiber eaten each day, the risk of heart disease decreased by 10 percent. This is equivalent to one portion of whole grains plus a portion of beans or lentils, or two to four servings of fruit and vegetables.

An apple a day? Yes, the old proverb seems to be true—according to a British study, if everyone over age fifty in that country ate only one apple a day, it could prevent 8,500 deaths due to cardiovascular disease each year. In comparison, it was estimated that 9,400 deaths could be prevented if these same people took a daily dose of a statin. However, the authors estimated that taking the statins would lead to 1,200 excess cases of muscle damage, 200 cases of severe kidney disease, and 12,300 new diagnoses of type 2 diabetes each year.

Sugar and Refined Carbohydrates

Although sugar has long been associated with diabetes, obesity, and hypertension, new evidence suggests that getting more than 10 percent of your daily calories from added sugar—equivalent to drinking as little as one extra soft drink each day—can increase your risk of death from CVD by 30 percent. People getting 25 percent or more of their daily calories from sugar have nearly three times the risk.

Refined carbohydrates—desserts, white rice, breakfast cereals, and white bread—also increase the risk of CVD. In a study of more than 75,000 healthy middle-aged women, there was almost twice the risk of cardiovascular disease after ten years in those who ate the highest percentage of refined carbohydrates. Another study of more than 117,000 Chinese men and women had a similar result—those consuming the highest proportion of refined carbohydrates, primarily white rice, had nearly twice the incidence of CVD.

Exercise

Exercise is important in reducing heart disease for many reasons. Not only does it help to prevent obesity, but it also strengthens the heart muscle itself and helps the flow of blood through blood vessels. Fitness, as measured by a treadmill test, reduces the risk of heart disease and stroke, especially over the long term. In one study of more than 16,000 people, those with low fitness had nearly twice the risk of death from CVD over thirty years as those with high fitness.

On the other hand, a sedentary lifestyle increases the risk of heart disease as well as death from all causes. Another study reported a 64 percent increased risk of dying from heart disease in men who spent more than twenty-three hours each week watching TV or riding in a car, compared to those who spent ten hours or less. Fortunately, there is evidence that replacing sitting with light activities such as walking around for as little as two minutes every hour can reduce the risk of death by about one-third.

How much exercise is enough? Recommendations vary, but the consensus is that thirty minutes five times a week of moderate exercise—brisk walking, swimming, biking, even dancing—is enough to significantly reduce your risk of heart disease. Unfortunately, only one in three adults in the United States gets the recommended amount of physical activity each week.

Obesity

Sixty-six percent of US women and 75 percent of men are overweight or obese, according to a nationwide health survey. The definitions of overweight and obese are based on a measure called the body mass index (BMI) that is calculated by using your height and weight. (See www.bmi-calculator.net to calculate your BMI.) Someone with a BMI between 25 and 30 is considered to be overweight, while having a BMI of 30 or more is considered obese.

Obesity, which affects about 35 percent of US adults, is associated with an increase in several risk factors for CVD—hypertension, atherosclerosis, and diabetes. The apple shaped distribution of fat that many men, and some women, develop puts them at higher risk for heart disease than fat that is distributed in the hips, the so-called "pear shape." In one study, people with a normal BMI but central obesity—measured by the ratio of the abdomen compared to the hips—had an increased risk of heart disease compared to those with a BMI of 30 who had no central obesity.

The emphasis by physicians on lowering cholesterol levels instead of encouraging lifestyle modifications is a powerful contributing factor to the perception that drugs alone will prevent heart disease. In fact, when some people are taking statin drugs, they actually gain weight. This could be due to the false security—or wishful thinking—that these medications can compensate for poor dietary choices and a sedentary lifestyle. A study found that after ten years, statin users consumed about 200 calories more per day than when they first started taking them and had gained from six to eleven pounds. Over the same period of time, nonusers did not increase their calories or gain weight.

Smoking

Smokers have twice the risk of cardiovascular disease as nonsmokers. But it's never too late to stop—even long-term smokers can reduce their risk of heart disease by quitting. An interesting study demonstrated that long-term smokers aged sixty and over who quit smoking for at least five years were able to lower their risk of death from heart disease by one-third. Current smokers were likely to die from heart disease five and a half years earlier than nonsmokers, while former smokers died two years earlier. For those smoking a pack or more a day, deaths from heart disease occurred nearly seven years earlier.

Psychological Factors

Psychological factors, such as anxiety, depression, and chronic stress, are all associated with increased CVD and death. In a combined analysis of six different studies, high stress was associated with a 27 percent increase in coronary heart disease. To put this in perspective, the authors likened this to the equivalent of smoking five cigarettes per day. And in a fascinating analysis of studies about the ill effects of acute stress, the risk of heart attacks increased nearly fivefold in men within two hours after outbursts of anger.

Using drugs to treat depression to reduce cardiac events in heart attack patients has not been successful. However, in a study of 237 Swedish women with coronary heart disease, those randomized to group stress-reduction counseling had significantly fewer deaths compared with patients who did not receive counseling.

Reducing stress is not easy, especially if you are in a difficult job or marriage or suffering from economic hardship. Adequate sleep, exercise, and relaxation techniques—yoga, breathing techniques, meditation, mindfulness training—can all help to manage stress. Engaging in pleasant activities like listening to music, walking outside in nature, or having a massage can also be therapeutic. Many hospitals, senior centers, and community organizations offer classes in relaxation techniques and stress management.

LIFESTYLE FACTORS THAT PREVENT CVD

- Eighty percent of cardiovascular disease can be prevented by changes in diet, exercise, and smoking.
- A Mediterranean diet can reduce heart disease by as much or more than statins, even in high-risk patients.
- One extra soft drink per day can increase the risk of death from heart disease by 30 percent.
- More than twenty-three hours per week of being sedentary increases the risk of heart disease by more than 60 percent.
- Smoking doubles the risk of heart disease; stress increases it by more than 25 percent.

MANAGING HIGH CHOLESTEROL WITHOUT DRUGS

For those who are concerned about lowering their cholesterol levels, various natural interventions have been shown to lower LDL cholesterol by as much as 20 percent. Whether or not they actually reduce CVD is unclear. These include plant sterols and stanols—substances that occur naturally in small amounts in many grains, vegetables, fruits, legumes, nuts, and seeds. They have a similar biochemical structure to cholesterol and have been found to block its absorption from the digestive tract. Manufacturers have started adding sterols and stanols to foods such as margarine, fruit juice, and pastries.

Apple cider vinegar lowered cholesterol levels significantly in several laboratory studies of rats, although there are no studies of this in humans. Fish oils and high-fiber foods—such as oatmeal, beans, nuts, and soy protein—can reduce LDL levels. High doses of niacin, also known as vitamin B_3, lowered LDL cholesterol by as much as 10 percent in some studies and decreased deaths from heart disease over the course of fifteen years. Unfortunately, the side effects of niacin—severe flushing of the face and upper body—make it difficult for many people to use.

Red yeast rice, a traditional Chinese medicine that contains a natural statin, has been reported to lower LDL cholesterol by as much as 19 percent in patients unable to tolerate pharmaceutical statins. However, if the red yeast rice is not fermented correctly, the contaminant citrinin can be present, which is potentially toxic to the kidneys and may be cancer causing. In a survey of twelve commercially available red yeast rice products, one-third of them contained citrinin.

STATIN DRUGS TO LOWER CHOLESTEROL

Although some doctors and researchers question the role of cholesterol in heart disease, the vast majority still believe that lowering LDL cholesterol will reduce your risk of CVD. Statins, the main class of drugs prescribed to do this, inhibit cholesterol production in the liver. There are a few other types of drugs for lowering cholesterol, but they are seldom used.

There is little difference between the various statin drugs, other than their strength, which is measured by how much of a drop in LDL cholesterol they will cause. Rosuvastatin (*Crestor*) is the strongest—a 40-milligram dose will lower LDL cholesterol by up to 60 percent, far more than most people need. A stronger dose also is more likely to cause side effects, as we saw with Sandra in chapter 1. And a stronger dose does not necessarily mean it is more effective. The maximum strength of atorvastatin (*Lipitor*), 80 milligrams, can lower LDL by an average of 50 percent. A head-to-head study comparing people taking 40 milligrams of rosuvastatin with those taking 80 milligrams of atorvastatin found that these two medicines were equally effective in reducing the amount of plaque in arteries after two years of treatment. Other common statin drugs are simvastatin (*Zocor*), fluvastatin (*Lescol*), lovastatin (*Mevacor*), and pravastatin (*Pravachol*).

Statins and Preventing Heart Disease

While many studies show that statins reduce cholesterol levels, most of the studies suggesting that statins reduce the actual number of heart attacks, strokes, or deaths have been done in patients who are at high risk for cardiovascular disease. These are people who already have had a heart attack or stroke or who have certain risk factors such as cigarette smoking, high blood pressure, obesity, or a family history of heart disease.

Even people with risk factors for heart disease might not benefit from statin treatment. A randomized trial of nearly 2,900 adults aged sixty-five and older with high blood pressure and elevated lipid levels but no evidence of heart disease was carried out. Researchers found no significant differences in overall deaths or deaths from coronary heart disease in those taking a statin. In those aged seventy-five or older, there was an actual increase in overall deaths in those taking statins.

For people with known heart disease, it has been calculated that for every eighty-three people treated for five years with a statin one life will be saved, and for every thirty-nine people treated, one nonfatal heart attack will be prevented. One out of every one hundred of these people will develop diabetes.

But what about everyone else? Harvard researchers reported that for people without risk factors or a previous heart attack or stroke, statins did not significantly decrease the risk of serious illness or death. They reported that 140 of these people would have to be treated with statins for five years to prevent only one nonfatal heart attack. At the same time, the authors estimated that one out of every five people taking statin drugs would experience a side effect, which you will learn more about later in this chapter.

Official Statin Guidelines

Official statin guidelines have become a moving target. When I was in medical school, a total cholesterol below 240 mg/dL was considered acceptable, but over the years that was lowered to 220 and then to 200 by various advisory groups. Even today, the American Heart Association considers a total cholesterol of 200–240 to be "borderline."

In 2004, new guidelines made LDL cholesterol, rather than total cholesterol, the primary factor in deciding whether to prescribe statins. These guidelines were so stringent that millions more Americans were prescribed these drugs. Subsequently, it was reported that "of the nine members of the panel that wrote the guidelines, six had each received research grants, speaking honoraria, or consulting fees from at least three and in some cases all five of the manufacturers of statins; only one had no financial links at all."

Fast forward to November 2013, when a consortium of heart organizations came out with yet a new set of guidelines. Forget LDL, they now said. What is most important is your overall risk of heart attack in the next ten years, determined by an online calculator. You should take a statin, they advised, if your risk is 7.5 percent or more—that is, if there is a seven-and-a-half chance out of one hundred that you will have a heart attack in the next ten years. Using the results of the online calculator, upwards of 70 million Americans, *including almost everyone over age sixty-five*, should be taking these drugs, a huge boon to the companies that manufacture them.

I checked my own risk score with this new calculator, found at www.cvriskcalculator.com. It asked questions about age, gender, race, total and HDL cholesterol levels, blood pressure, diabetes, and smoking. I was surprised to find no questions about family history, obesity, diet, or exercise, since all of these also are associated with heart disease. The verdict came—*you have a 5.5 percent risk of heart attack or stroke in the next ten years*. Whew. But when I changed my age from sixty-four to sixty-eight, my risk increased to 7.9 percent and I was advised to take a statin.

These new guidelines have caused considerable controversy. Many doctors still believe that LDL cholesterol should be the major factor when deciding whether to prescribe a statin. Some think that the 7.5 percent risk parameter is too strict and should be changed to 20 percent, which is used in the United Kingdom. The validity of the actual calculator has been called into question, since it is based on twenty-year-old data. One analysis reported that the calculator overestimated the risk of cardiovascular events by 83 percent in men and 67 percent in women. Another drawback—the calculator is based on values measured only once, not giving an accurate picture of day-to-day fluctuations in blood pressure and cholesterol levels.

Earlier guidelines recommended that "therapeutic lifestyle changes—low saturated fat and low cholesterol diet, physical activity, and weight control—remain the *cornerstone of treatment* for lowering cholesterol levels." The newest guidelines are solely focused on taking statins, with no mention of recommendations for lifestyle changes.

CHOLESTEROL AND STATIN FACTS

- Cholesterol is found in every cell of the body and is an essential building block for the production of hormones, vitamin D, and other compounds.
- Seventy-two percent of people admitted to the hospital with a first heart attack did not have high cholesterol.
- Statins, the most widely used drugs in the United States, block the production of cholesterol in the liver.
- More than half of all men and 40 percent of all women over age sixty-five take statins.
- One hundred and forty healthy people would need to take statins for five years to prevent one heart attack.
- Statin guidelines overestimate the risk for heart disease by 83 percent in men and 67 percent in women.

STATIN SIDE EFFECTS

Almost one in five patients stop taking statins due to unacceptable side effects. These include muscle pain, memory problems, diabetes, cataracts, liver and kidney failure, mood disorders, and possibly suicide.

Muscle Damage

Muscle damage, or myopathy, is the most common adverse effect of statins. A European panel reported that 7 to 29 percent of statin users had muscle symptoms—weakness, aches, and pains—the most common reason that people stop taking them. Statin users, especially those who are physically active, are more likely to have injuries such as sprains, strains, and dislocations. A less common but much more dangerous side effect of statins is rhabdomyolysis, a serious muscle injury that can lead to kidney failure and death.

Scientists studying muscle tissues in rats found that those given *Lipitor* showed nearly twice as much muscle damage after running on a treadmill than those who were not taking any drugs. The muscle pain and weakness of people taking statins may cause them to exercise less or not at all. And, as we know, lack of exercise is a risk factor for heart disease. Statins also can impair the functioning of the heart muscle itself.

The muscle side effects of statins appear to be dose related— the higher the dose of statin taken, the more chance there is of muscle damage. Since statins, like most other medicines, are usually prescribed in the same dosage to everyone, a small woman is often given the same dose as a much larger man. This will lead to a higher concentration of the drug in her bloodstream and a higher risk of side effects. Taking statins along with other medications, including certain antibiotics, antidepressants, cardiovascular drugs, and even quinine, can nearly double the risk of muscle injury. Examples of these drugs include amiodarone (*Cordarone*), cimetidine (*Tagamet*), ciprofloxacin (*Cipro*), and paroxetine (*Paxil*).

Ted, a retired fireman, loved to sail his 42-foot ketch on Puget Sound. His wife, Gloria, was a retired emergency department nurse who wrote articles for the local boating magazine. One day, Ted noticed a pulling pain in his left calf after walking the short distance from his car to the boat. He thought this was strange, since he didn't remember doing anything to hurt it. The pain continued for the rest of the day and became worse that night. Over the next few days the pain became so bad that Ted couldn't walk.

Gloria finally persuaded him to see their family doctor, who took a brief history and ordered some tests. All the results came back normal. The doctor was baffled about what was causing this pain. Then she looked at Ted's medication chart and noticed that he had recently started taking a statin to lower his cholesterol. "Bingo!" she said. Explaining that statins sometimes cause muscle pain, she recommended that he stop taking it. Within forty-eight hours the pain had subsided and Ted decided to forgo further statin treatment. His cholesterol had been in the borderline range, 210, and he planned to bring it down using diet and exercise.

Memory Loss and Dementia

The most disturbing side effects of statins are those that affect the mind. Statins block the production of cholesterol, which is important in transmitting messages from one brain cell to another. Since one-fourth of the body's cholesterol is found in the brain, it is not surprising that statins can cause problems with mental functioning.

In 2012, the FDA issued a safety announcement cautioning that cognitive problems—memory loss, forgetfulness, amnesia, memory impairment, and confusion—may be associated with statin use and urged patients to tell their doctors if they experienced any of these symptoms. The report advised that these symptoms can occur after taking a statin for only one day or after taking them for several years. In a survey of statin patients who experienced cognitive problems, 90 percent of them improved when they stopped taking the drug. There were more cognitive side effects in those taking higher dose statins.

Herbert was a Harvard history professor who was having problems remembering the names of his students and keeping up with his professional correspondence. He was diagnosed with Alzheimer's disease after he gradually lost the ability to recognize people he knew or to remember more than one page he read at a time.

When Herbert decided to participate in a study of a new Alzheimer's drug, his statin drug was discontinued prior to starting the study and, unexpectedly, his mental functioning began to improve. He was excluded from the study after it was determined that he no longer qualified. After he stopped taking the statin, he slowly began to regain more and more of his memory, but it took two full years for his mental capacity to return to normal.

The most compelling evidence about the effect of statins on memory loss is from a study looking at nearly a million patients who were followed for more than twenty-five years. Those who were taking statins had four times the risk of experiencing acute memory loss within the first thirty days of taking them compared to people who were not taking them. More evidence of the importance of cholesterol for proper brain function—a study of people aged seventy and above found that *those with the highest cholesterol levels had the least risk of dementia.*

The Alzheimer's Association estimates that one in ten people aged sixty-five and older in the United States has this disease. By 2050, they estimate the number of people with Alzheimer's will triple—from more than five million to sixteen million people, each one with a family that is burdened financially and emotionally. The total cost to the health-care system in 2017 for this illness is estimated to be $259 billion—more than a quarter of a trillion dollars. There was an 89 percent increase in deaths from Alzheimer's between 2000 and 2014.

Unfortunately, none of the large clinical trials of statins for heart disease have looked at mental functioning, nor have there been clinical studies comparing cognitive loss in statin users to those taking a placebo. Given the importance of cholesterol in brain functioning, the large number of people taking statins, the growing incidence of Alzheimer's disease, and reports of cognitive problems reversing after discontinuing statin therapy, it is vital that more research is done on this subject.

Type 2 Diabetes

Evidence is mounting that statins increase the risk of type 2—adult-onset—diabetes. People with type 2 diabetes have higher than normal blood sugar levels because their bodies don't properly use or produce enough insulin. Researchers suspect that statins impair insulin secretion and inhibit insulin release from cells. The FDA mandated a labeling change for statins to alert patients about the increased diabetes risk, in the same 2012 announcement that warned of cognitive problems.

Data from the Women's Health Initiative (WHI), a twenty-five-year study of almost 162,000 postmenopausal women, showed that women on all types of statin drugs had a 48 percent increased risk of developing diabetes. Those who were not overweight had an even higher risk, perhaps due to their smaller body size. Another study followed more than 8,700 nondiabetic patients for nearly six years. Those taking statins had a 46 percent increased risk of developing type 2 diabetes and those taking higher dose statins had an even higher risk.

Even more troubling is a study that matched healthy statin users with nonusers. There was a nearly twofold increase in developing new-onset diabetes and more than double the risk of diabetic complications in those taking statins. Those on the highest dose statins had the highest risks. There is no longer any doubt that the risk of diabetes in statin users is considerable.

Dennis, a sixty-two-year-old former construction worker, had gained sixty pounds since he retired. His waist size had gone from 34 to 42 inches. He also smoked at least one pack of cigarettes a day. During his annual checkup, his cholesterol level was too high—285. His doctor told Dennis that unless he changed his habits, he was a prime candidate for a heart attack or stroke and urged him to lose weight and stop smoking.

Dennis said he would prefer to take a pill, so his doctor prescribed *Lipitor*. Dennis was happy to take this while he continued to smoke and eat a high-fat diet. Unfortunately, he was recently diagnosed with diabetes and is now taking medication to treat that too.

Cataracts and Macular Degeneration

The development of cataracts, a clouding of the lens of the eye, is another disturbing side effect of statins. Data from a large military health-care system showed a 27 percent increased risk of cataracts in those taking statins, while a Canadian study found a 48 percent increased risk of cataracts in statin users. Macular degeneration, another age-related eye disease associated with blindness, has also been associated with statin use.

Other Adverse Effects

A British study found that statin users have one and a half times the risk of moderate or severe liver damage compared to nonusers, with the severity of the problem being dose related. The FDA recommends that liver function be tested in all patients before starting statins and that patients be alert for signs of liver problems, such as dark urine or yellowing of the skin or eyes. The same British study reported that statin users also have a one and a half to two times greater risk of kidney failure, especially those taking high-dose formulations. This risk appeared within the first year of treatment and persisted over the next five years. Even after statins were discontinued, it took a full year for the risk of kidney failure to return to normal.

Researchers estimate that excessive fatigue affects between 20 and 40 percent of patients taking statins. In a randomized trial of more than 1,000 patients with elevated LDL levels, half were given a statin and the others received a look-alike placebo. After six months, there was a significant increase in overall tiredness as well as post-exercise fatigue in those who were taking the statin. And according to another study, statin users have a 30 percent increased risk of back disorders, including herniated discs and spinal stenosis—narrowing of the open spaces in the spine. Low cholesterol has been found to be related to several types of mood disorders and even suicide. There is preliminary evidence of other side effects associated with statins, including sexual dysfunction, aggressive behavior, gastrointestinal problems, skin rashes, sleep disorders, and autoimmune diseases.

STATIN SIDE EFFECTS

- One in five patients taking statins have side effects, muscle pain is the most common.
- The FDA has issued safety announcements cautioning statin users about memory problems, diabetes, and liver function.
- Acute memory loss is four times more common in statin users in the first thirty days of treatment.
- People taking statins have nearly a 50 percent higher risk of developing type 2 diabetes.
- Other side effects include cataracts, liver and kidney damage, fatigue, back pain and mood disorders.

DO YOU REALLY NEED THAT STATIN PILL?

In making the decision about whether or not to take a statin, you should weigh your risk of heart disease against the possible side effects of the medication. The new guidelines, which many think are faulty, recommend a statin if your risk of having a heart attack or stroke in the next ten years is 7.5 percent. That means you have a 92.5 percent chance of not having one. Keep in mind also that one out of every five people taking statins experiences side effects, some of them very serious.

If you have had a previous heart attack or stroke and/or if you have a 20 percent risk of having one in the next ten years using the British calculator (qrisk.org), you should consider taking statins *if you are not able to reduce your ten-year risk using lifestyle methods alone.* In people with familial hypercholesterolemia, a genetic defect causing high levels of LDL cholesterol, statins are usually recommended.

If you do opt to take a statin, take the lowest dose necessary to keep your total cholesterol level below 220 mg/dL. This is true especially for women, who are more vulnerable to the side effects of statins owing to their smaller size. Be aware of possible side effects while taking statins and consult your medical provider at the first sign of any problem. Supplementation with coenzyme Q10 can alleviate the muscle pains associated with statins but it is not known if this supplement can alleviate any of the other side effects.

While it is easier to take a pill, most of us could take a thirty-minute walk three times a week, up our intake of fruits and vegetables to five servings daily, and cut down on highly refined carbohydrates. Losing weight and stopping smoking are more difficult but can be done with proper motivation and support. Given the choice, which would you do? Change your lifestyle or take a pill? As the evidence of serious side effects from statins continues to grow—diabetes, cataracts, muscle damage, even dementia—the risk benefit equation tilts dramatically toward not taking them at all.

Chapter 4

Osteoporosis

If you are a woman over age sixty-five, chances are you've been tested for osteoporosis. This is because, since the mid-1990s, scans have become available to measure bone density. Before that, the diagnosis of osteoporosis was extremely rare, made only after a broken bone. Seventy percent of people over age eighty worldwide are now said to have osteoporosis. But this is not surprising, since the diagnosis of osteoporosis is made by comparing someone's bone density, which all of us lose as we age, to that of a thirty-year-old. In the meantime, routine testing for bone density has turned this condition into a gold mine for companies selling drugs to thwart the condition. The worldwide market for osteoporosis drugs is estimated to reach $9 billion by 2020.

WHAT IS OSTEOPOROSIS?

In the simplest of terms, osteoporosis is the gradual thinning of bones. It happens as people age because the breakdown of bone tissue by cells called *osteoclasts* happens faster than bone can be built back up by other cells, *osteoblasts*. This is in contrast to the buildup of bone mass that occurs until around age thirty. Osteoporosis is more common after menopause due to lack of estrogen, which protects bone mass. It is more often found in Caucasians and Asians than in African Americans or Hispanics and in those who are small and thin, as well as in people with a family history of osteoporosis.

Because osteoporosis causes bones to become thin and brittle, they tend to break more easily. The most likely places they break are the hip, spine, and wrist. Usually this is the result of an injury but sometimes bones break spontaneously, especially in the spine. Elderly people who are permanently bent forward are usually suffering from osteoporosis of the spine. Oftentimes there are no symptoms of osteoporosis until someone breaks a bone, although a loss of height and/or the development of a small curvature in the upper spine are clues that it might be a problem.

Measuring Bone Density

The DEXA scan (dual-energy X-ray absorptiometry), a noninvasive low-energy X-ray evaluation of the hip, wrist, and spine, was first used in 1994 to establish the diagnosis of osteoporosis. This was done by a World Health Organization (WHO) study group that received financial support from several pharmaceutical companies, as well as from a private nonprofit foundation. Results of this scan are reported as a T-score, a comparison to the bone density that is typically found in a thirty-year-old woman. A T-score of 0 to -1 is considered normal, while someone with a score of less than -2.5 is diagnosed with osteoporosis. Someone with a bone density between -1 and -2.5 is said to have *osteopenia*, a disorder defined solely by the results of the DEXA scan. Based on these definitions, almost 44 percent of US adults aged fifty years and older have osteopenia, while slightly more than 10 percent have osteoporosis.

The first drugs to treat osteoporosis came out in 1995, shortly after this disorder was defined by the DEXA scan. Since then, a web-based tool (FRAX) that predicts your risk of a hip fracture has been introduced by a similar WHO group to identify those who might benefit from pharmaceutical treatment. Using the FRAX calculator, almost three-fourths of US women over age sixty-five and nearly 95 percent of women over age seventy-five are diagnosed as needing drug treatment.

While most doctors rely on the results of the DEXA scan to diagnose osteoporosis, the test itself is not recommended for women under age sixty-five and most men, according to the American Board of Internal Medicine (ABIM). Even in women over sixty-five, having the test exposes you to radiation as well as the risk of being diagnosed with osteopenia and being put on drugs with risky side effects. Although the amount of radiation is small, it can add up over the years.

Osteoporosis and Hip Fractures

The main reason given for treating osteoporosis is to prevent hip fractures, a major cause of disability and death. Twenty to thirty percent of people with hip fractures die within one year and about 50 percent are unable to live independently afterward. But recent evidence has called into question whether osteoporosis is the primary cause of hip fractures and whether osteoporosis drugs are effective in preventing them.

In a groundbreaking analysis published in the top-ranking *British Medical Journal (BMJ)* in 2015, researchers from six different countries defied conventional medical thought about bone fractures and osteoporosis. They questioned the current assumption that fragile bones, as measured by the DEXA scan or risk calculator, predict hip fractures and that drug treatment will prevent these fractures. They pointed out that:

- Fewer than one in three hip fractures are the result of fragile bones; most are in people without osteoporosis.
- Impaired balance is a better predictor of hip fractures than osteoporosis.
- One hundred seventy-five postmenopausal women with osteoporosis must be treated with drugs for three years to prevent one hip fracture.
- Although osteoporosis is considered primarily a disease of females, 30 to 40 percent of hip fractures occur in men.
- Exercise has been found to reduce the risk of falling by as much as 60 percent.
- Reliance on pharmaceutical treatments for osteoporosis prevents people from making lifestyle modifications and exercising to keep their bones healthy.

PREVENTING OSTEOPOROSIS WITHOUT DRUGS

Even if osteoporosis is not the major contributor to hip fractures, it is still advisable to do all you can to prevent bone loss. If you do fall, your bones are more likely to break if they are fragile. Whether or not you develop osteoporosis and how severe it becomes depends on many factors, including your genes, lifestyle, and where you live. While attributes like race and genetic makeup cannot be altered, there are several things you can do to keep your bones healthy and reduce your risk of osteoporosis. Many people are able to avoid this condition well into their eighties by paying attention to several important factors.

Calcium

A lifelong diet rich in calcium can help you avoid osteoporosis. Bones are made up primarily of calcium, so you need to make sure your body has enough of this important building block. Calcium is also needed for many other bodily processes, such as blood clotting and the functioning of muscles and nerves. If you don't consume enough calcium, it will be taken from your bones.

The recommended daily amount of calcium is 1,000 milligrams if you are under age fifty and 1,200 milligrams if you are older than that. You probably already know that dairy products—milk, cheese, and yogurt—are a good source of calcium. Other calcium-rich foods include dark-green leafy vegetables, such as broccoli, collard greens, kale, and spinach, as well as sardines and salmon with bones, tofu, and almonds.

Calcium Supplements

The best source of calcium is from your food, so you should try to meet your daily requirement from diet alone. If you are not able to do this, consider taking a calcium supplement. Experts at an international meeting about osteoporosis recommended calcium and vitamin D supplements for people at risk for this disease. They also concluded that there is no increased risk of heart disease from taking calcium, a previous concern. The National Osteoporosis Foundation recommends calcium supplements for women over age fifty and others at increased risk.

If you do decide to take a supplement, check the label to find out how much *elemental* calcium is in each dose. Take enough to equal, along with food sources, the recommended daily amount for your age. More than this is not needed and too much can cause gas and constipation. Calcium supplements should be taken with food since the body needs stomach acid to digest them. It is better to take them two to three times a day instead of all at once. Vitamin D is needed to absorb calcium, so many supplements combine these two into one tablet.

Vitamin D

Even if you consume enough calcium, your body cannot absorb it without vitamin D. You can get vitamin D from two sources—food and sunlight. Foods that are high in vitamin D include egg yolks, fatty fish such as salmon and sardines, and dairy products that are vitamin D fortified. Cod liver oil is high in vitamin D. Most experts recommend a daily intake of 800 to 1,000 international units (IU) of vitamin D to reach optimal blood levels.

Humans have the wonderful capacity to transform the energy of the sun into vitamin D. Sun exposure can produce up to 3,000 IU of vitamin D per day depending on the amount of the body exposed, the strength or angle of the sun, and skin color. Those living in higher latitudes with little or no sun in the winter months are often deficient in vitamin D, which explains why hip fractures are more common in Scandinavia and North America.

If you live in North America and have light to medium colored skin, spending a total of one hour each week outside in the sun with your arms exposed and *without sunscreen* will give you adequate amounts of vitamin D. Those with darker skin need more time. However, sunscreen will block it—a product with a 30 SPF reduces the production of vitamin D by 97 percent.

You might be concerned about the risk of skin cancer if you don't use sunscreen. A total of one hour each week spread over several days is not dangerous. Most people don't realize that the most common forms of skin cancer—squamous and basal cell—are not life-threatening and rarely spread beyond the surface of the skin.

The type of skin cancer that *is* dangerous is melanoma, which can spread internally to vital organs and become fatal. While long-term sun exposure can lead to the more harmless types of skin cancer, melanoma is thought to be the result of a brief, intense exposure to the sun, such as a blistering sunburn, rather than years of mild exposure.

Risks of Low Vitamin D Levels

Having a low vitamin D level is dangerous and increases the risk of cancer, heart disease, and dementia. A provocative study of over 30,000 Swedish women reported that avoiding the sun was as much of a risk factor for death as smoking. The life expectancy of those who avoided the sun was as much as two years shorter than those who had the highest sun exposure.

Data from ninety-five different studies which included nearly one million people revealed that those with the lowest levels of vitamin D were 35 percent more likely to die from heart disease, 15 percent more likely to die from cancer, and 30 percent more likely to die from all other causes. Elderly patients with vitamin D deficiency are more likely to have a decline in their mental functioning. Age-related macular degeneration (AMD), a leading cause of blindness in older adults, has been associated with low vitamin D levels as well.

Vitamin D Supplements

Because there are so few food sources of vitamin D and many people do not get enough from the sun, supplementation is often needed. A blood serum level of 40 to 50 nanograms/milliliter (ng/mL) of 25-hydroxy vitamin D—25(OH)D—is the optimum value for preventing osteoporosis and other chronic diseases. This is not measured in routine blood tests, but you can request that your doctor order it. If your 25(OH)D is not high enough and you cannot increase it from food or the sun, consider taking a vitamin D supplement.

The amount of supplemental vitamin D needed varies from person to person. The Endocrine Society recommends 800 IU per day of vitamin D_3 to maintain an adequate blood level. If your level is low, you might need to take 1,000 to 2,000 IU daily for several months to bring it up to an acceptable value. Taking a supplement for two to three months and then rechecking your 25(OH)D level will help you determine if your dosage is sufficient. There is very little danger of overdosing with vitamin D if you are taking less than 4,000 IU per day.

Exercise

Because bones are living tissue, exercise can strengthen them, much as exercise strengthens muscles. And exercise can reduce the risk of falls and hip fractures. Several different types of exercise are important in maintaining bone health:

- Weight-bearing exercises—these are exercises in which your body moves against gravity. They include walking, dancing, hiking, jogging, and playing tennis.
- Resistance exercises—these involve strengthening your muscles. They include activities like weight lifting, exercising with elastic bands, and using weight machines.
- Nonimpact exercises—these help to improve balance and posture and can help prevent falls leading to broken bones. Yoga, Pilates, and tai chi are examples of these.

Before beginning a new exercise program, make sure you consult your medical provider.

Smoking, Alcohol, and Caffeine

Smoking decreases bone mass and causes an increase in fractures, although the exact reason is not well understood. Moderation seems to be the key as far as alcohol and caffeine are concerned. More than two drinks per day can decrease bone density and increase the risk of bone fractures. Large amounts of caffeine (more than eighteen ounces of brewed coffee per day) have been reported to accelerate bone loss in postmenopausal women.

Carbonated Soft Drinks

There has been concern for several years about the connection between carbonated soft drinks and osteoporosis. A study published in 2006 found that cola drinks can decrease bone density. More recently, a thirty-year study of nearly 75,000 postmenopausal women reported that for every soft drink consumed in a day, there was a 15 percent increased risk of hip fracture. This was true for all soft drinks—those with and without caffeine, diet and regular sodas, and colas versus noncolas. One reason for this could be that phosphoric acid in sodas can leach calcium from bones. Or it may happen because soft drinks sometimes take the place of more healthy calcium-containing drinks such as milk. Seltzers and soda water do not contain phosphoric acid and have not been reported to contribute to osteoporosis.

Medications That Increase the Risk of Osteoporosis

There are several classes of drugs that can increase your risk of osteoporosis. Minimizing the use of them will help keep your bones healthy.

Steroid drugs such as prednisone can cause osteoporosis by inhibiting the production of bone tissue and increasing its breakdown, which decreases overall bone mass. Studies have found a correlation between steroids, used by 2.5 percent of people ages seventy to seventy-nine, and fracture risk, even with low doses. Anyone taking them for more than three months should take supplemental calcium and vitamin D and make sure they are getting plenty of weight-bearing exercise.

Proton pump inhibitors (PPIs) for acid reflux interfere with the absorption of calcium in the stomach, which can lead to thinning of bones. Several studies have shown that older women taking PPIs have an increased risk of hip or spine fractures. Selective serotonin reuptake inhibitor (SSRI) antidepressants can double the risk of bone fractures. When taken by postmenopausal women, SSRIs were found to cause an even higher risk of fractures than steroids or PPIs. Other drugs associated with increased risk of fractures or decreased bone mass include thiazolidinedione diabetes drugs (*Avandia and Actos*), antiepileptic drugs, and anticoagulants like warfarin (*Coumadin*).

Preventing Falls

Osteoporosis itself is not always a problem. The main danger is having brittle bones that can break easily if you fall. Reducing your chance of falling is an important part of lowering the risks from osteoporosis. Half of the twenty most commonly prescribed medications taken by older adults may increase the risk of falls. Some commonsense measures to reduce your risk of falls are:

- Do exercises that improve balance and increase lower body strength.
- Remove clutter from hallways and stairs.
- Wear sensible shoes that grip the floor; avoid flip-flops and slippers with slippery soles.

- Have your vision checked regularly.
- Remove throw rugs or secure them to the floor with double-sided tape.
- Install handrails in the shower and along staircases.
- Install nonslip strips in the shower.
- Avoid medications that can make you dizzy, like tranquilizers, sedatives, opioid painkillers, and antidepressants.

MEDICATIONS TO TREAT OSTEOPOROSIS

Osteoporosis occurs when the amount of bone being removed is greater than that being produced, leading to a net loss. Treatment approaches include those that slow down the removal of bone, and those that work by increasing bone production.

Bisphosphonates

Bisphosphonates are the most common medications used to treat osteoporosis. Common ones are: alendronate (*Fosamax*), risedronate (*Actonel*), ibandronate (*Boniva*), and zoledronate (*Reclast*). These drugs slow the breakdown of bone tissue by osteoclasts. Overall bone density increases since bone is still being made at the same rate while bone is being lost more slowly. The problem with these drugs is that old bone tissue is not being cleared away in order to make room for new growth. While bone density might look better on X-ray exams after taking these drugs, the actual bone that is there is older and more likely to break.

There is little evidence that bisphosphonates are effective in strengthening bones and preventing fractures. A Canadian study found no difference in the incidence of hip fractures across several provinces, even though four times as many women took osteoporosis medication in some of the provinces compared to the others. Another study of the risk of hip fractures in women aged sixty-five and over found no difference between those who took bisphosphonates and those who did not. Even more stunning was the finding that those who took the drugs for more than three years had a 33 percent *increased* risk of hip fracture compared to those who had never taken them.

Fosamax and *Actonel* are taken daily, weekly, or monthly and are sometimes combined into one tablet with vitamin D_3 or calcium. Due to a tendency to cause an upset stomach, they should be taken on an empty stomach with a glass of water. It is important to stay upright—sitting, standing, or walking—for at least thirty minutes after taking them. *Boniva* is taken once a month as a tablet or every three months by intravenous (IV) injection, while *Reclast* is given intravenously once yearly.

Side Effects of Bisphosphonates

Bisphosphonates can be difficult to tolerate. Gastrointestinal symptoms of the oral tablets include nausea, heartburn, difficulty swallowing, irritation of the esophagus, and stomach ulcers. In addition, the FDA cautions doctors about "the possibility of severe and sometimes incapacitating bone, joint, and/or muscle (musculoskeletal) pain in patients taking bisphosphonates. . . . Pain may occur within days, months, or years after starting a bisphosphonate." Side effects of the IV infusions include flulike symptoms that can last two to three days with fever, headache, and muscle or joint pain. Up to 20 percent of people stop taking bisphosphonates due to these problems.

Fractures of the Thigh Bones

In 2010, the FDA issued a safety announcement alerting doctors to the risk of an unusual kind of spontaneous fracture of the thigh bone in those taking bisphosphonates for more than five years. The latest research suggests that these fractures are related to microscopic cracks that develop from suppressing the removal of old bone tissue by osteoclasts.

Thigh pain is a warning sign that often occurs before the bone breaks. There is evidence that the longer one takes these medications the greater the risk. It is estimated that one out of 1,000 long-term users will have this problem each year. Many experts advise that women stop taking bisphosphonates after five years.

Necrosis of the Jaw

Another rare but serious long-term effect of taking bisphosphonates is necrosis (dead tissue) of the jawbone. This typically occurs after dental work and can cause abscesses, teeth to fall out, and even the eating away of the tissues of the cheek, exposing the jaw bone. While this complication is mostly seen in cancer patients being treated with IV formulations of bisphosphonates, an increased risk of necrosis of the jaw has also been reported in those taking oral medications.

Atrial Fibrillation

In an analysis of twelve different studies, researchers reported an increased risk of atrial fibrillation in 25 to 40 percent of bisphosphonate users. Atrial fibrillation is a rapid and irregular heartbeat that increases the risk of blood clots and strokes.

Esophageal Cancer

Finally, there is some evidence that bisphosphonates may increase the risk of esophageal cancer, perhaps due to chronic irritation. In an analysis of seven studies of nearly 20,000 cases of esophageal cancer, those taking bisphosphonates had a significantly higher risk for it. Those who had been taking them for more than three years had more than twice the risk than those taking them for less than one year. Another analysis found no significant risk of esophageal cancer but the authors cautioned that with such a rare disease, very large studies with sufficiently long follow-up would be needed to adequately assess the risk.

Other Medications for Osteoporosis

Because of the risks of taking bisphosphonates, several other medicines have been introduced to treat osteoporosis. Most of these have been shown to reduce fractures of the spine but not the hip and are prescribed for people who are at increased risk of fractures, such as those who have previously had one.

Raloxifene (*Evista*) is in a class of drugs called SERMS (selective estrogen receptor modulators). It was developed to mimic the bone-enhancing effects of estrogen, which stimulates osteoblasts to produce new bone. It also has antiestrogen effects on the uterus, reducing the cancer risk that comes with excessive estrogen. Its most common side effects come from both the estrogen effects—blood clots in the legs and the lungs, and the antiestrogen effects—hot flashes and other menopausal symptoms. It is approved only for postmenopausal women. Raloxifene has been found to decrease the risk of breast cancer in postmenopausal women but it also increases the risk of having a fatal stroke.

Teriparatide (*Forteo*) is a genetically engineered form of the naturally occurring parathyroid hormone that increases the activity of osteoblasts, which build up bone mass. It is given by a daily self-injection under the skin. Side effects include dizziness, depression, nausea, vomiting, constipation, and fatigue. It increases the amount of calcium in the bloodstream as well as uric acid and can cause a sudden drop in blood pressure after injections, leading to the recommendation that it be taken sitting down.

Denosumab (*Prolia*) is a human antibody produced in the laboratory that inactivates osteoclasts, slowing the breakdown of bone tissue. It is injected under the skin once every six months and is approved only for people at high risk of bone fractures when other osteoporosis medications haven't worked. Side effects include headache, muscle and joint pain, nausea, diarrhea, back pain, and many more serious ones.

Type of Osteoporosis Medication	Examples (Brand Name)	How They Work	Possible Side Effects
Bisphosphonates	Alendronate (*Fosamax*); Risedronate (*Actonel*); Ibandronate (*Boniva*); Zoledronate (*Reclast*)	Slow the breakdown of bone tissue by osteoclasts	Nausea, heartburn, difficulty swallowing, irritation of the esophagus, and stomach ulcers; bone, joint, and muscle pain; flulike symptoms; fracture of the thigh bone; necrosis of the jaw bone; atrial fibrillation; esophageal cancer

Selective estrogen receptor modulators (SERMS)	Raloxifene (*Evista*)	Mimic the bone enhancing effects of estrogen, stimulating osteoblasts to produce new bone	Blood clots in the legs and lungs, hot flashes, and other menopausal symptoms
Genetically engineered parathyroid hormone	Teriparatide (*Forteo*)	Increases the activity of osteoblasts, which build up bone mass	Dizziness, depression, nausea, vomiting, constipation, and fatigue
Lab-created human antibody	Denosumab (*Prolia*)	Inactivates osteoclasts, slowing breakdown of bone tissue	Headache, muscle and joint pain, nausea, diarrhea, and back pain

DO YOU REALLY NEED THAT OSTEOPOROSIS PILL?

The evidence for the effectiveness of osteoporosis medications in preventing hip and other fractures is questionable and their side effects are considerable. Whether or not to take them depends on a variety of factors, including your age, gender, and medical history.

There is little evidence that these drugs are helpful or cost-effective for people with mild bone loss. If you are diagnosed with osteopenia, you are much better off concentrating on the things that will keep your bones healthy, such as making sure you have enough calcium and vitamin D as well as exercising regularly. The same can be true if you have been diagnosed with osteoporosis, although concentrating on fall prevention is especially important for you.

If you have had a previous hip or spine fracture or have certain other risk factors, you might consider taking an osteoporosis medication. Such risk factors include breaking a bone in a minor accident, having a parent who broke a hip, smoking, drinking heavily, having a low body weight, having rheumatoid arthritis (RA), or taking corticosteroids for more than three months.

As the authors of the 2015 *BMJ* analysis on osteoporosis and hip fractures concluded: "The dominant approach to hip fracture prevention is neither viable as a public health strategy nor cost effective. Pharmacotherapy can achieve at best a marginal reduction in hip fractures at the cost of unnecessary psychological harms, serious medical adverse events, and forgone opportunities to have greater impacts on the health of older people. As such, it is an intellectual fallacy we will live to regret."

Chapter 5

Acid Reflux Disease

Do you suffer from heartburn or indigestion? Have you been told that you have acid reflux, also known as gastroesophageal reflux disease (GERD)? If so, it is likely that you have been told to take a proton pump inhibitor (PPI). Thirteen billion dollars are spent each year on these drugs in the United States, while some medical experts say that up to seven out of ten people are taking them inappropriately. The PPI *Nexium* was the fourth leading prescription drug in the United States for the twelve-month period ending in March 2015, with fifteen million prescriptions and sales topping $5 billion. Nearly one out of every five people aged sixty-two and over take a PPI.

These numbers are truly staggering, especially in light of the growing list of serious potential long-term problems attributed to PPIs. Dementia, vitamin deficiencies, fractures, pneumonia, chronic kidney disease, and dangerous gastrointestinal infections are some of the complications of PPIs that have been reported in medical journals. And the majority of people who are taking them are doing so needlessly.

WHAT IS ACID REFLUX?

Upward of 15 million Americans suffer daily from acid reflux, while 60 million people experience symptoms at least once a month. Despite what you might think, acid reflux is *not* caused by excess stomach acid. It is caused by a weakness in the muscle—the lower esophageal sphincter—that opens to let food from the esophagus into the stomach and then closes to stop food and stomach acids from coming back up into the esophagus. If the muscle doesn't close properly, food and acids come back up and irritate the lining of the esophagus, causing bleeding and other serious complications.

Symptoms of acid reflux include burning in the chest behind the breastbone, nausea, and regurgitation of fluids into the mouth with a bitter or acid taste—called water brash. Coughing, hoarseness, sore throat, and a feeling of a lump in the throat are other symptoms. Chest pain can be so severe that it is confused with a heart attack. Sometimes the upper part of the stomach protrudes into the chest cavity, causing a hiatal hernia, increasing the risk of acid reflux. Obesity, pregnancy, cigarette smoking, asthma, and diabetes are all risk factors for developing this disorder.

Symptoms similar to acid reflux can also be caused by an infection with a bacteria, *Helicobacter pylori*, that causes no symptoms in many people but causes stomach irritation and peptic ulcers in others. *Helicobacter* should be diagnosed and treated with antibiotics rather than medicine for acid reflux.

MANAGING ACID REFLUX WITHOUT DRUGS

Doctors can be quick to recommend medication for acid reflux. But before popping that pill, especially if you have only occasional problems, try some commonsense and natural ways to alleviate your symptoms.

Commonsense Methods to Treat Acid Reflux

There are several simple commonsense methods that can help reduce your symptoms of acid reflux:

- Lose weight. Sometimes only five or ten pounds is enough to make a difference.
- Avoid tight clothing around your waist—this puts added pressure on your stomach.
- Avoid mint, garlic, onion, tomato sauce, fatty or fried foods, chocolate, caffeine, and alcohol, all of which can cause heartburn.
- Stop smoking, which relaxes the lower esophageal sphincter, allowing acids to move upward.
- Eat several small meals throughout the day to reduce the amount of food in your stomach at any one time.
- Wait two to three hours after dinner before going to bed. This allows food to move past your stomach before you lie down.
- Elevate the head of your bed by six to eight inches or add a wedge under your mattress to help gravity keep food in your stomach where it belongs.

Heartburn can be a side effect of many drugs, including antidepressants, anxiety medications, antibiotics, blood pressure medications, nitroglycerin, and osteoporosis drugs. Check the package inserts of any medications you are taking or ask your pharmacist if they might be causing your symptoms. If so, ask your doctor to reduce your dosage or prescribe something else.

Patricia, an intensive care nurse, had gradually put on an extra twenty-five pounds, mostly around her abdomen. She was so tired when she got home from work that she mostly watched TV and didn't exercise. One night, she awoke from a sound sleep with heartburn so intense that she could hardly breathe. Stomach acids were coming up into her esophagus and causing her throat to spasm. She had to sit up in bed for two hours before the burning in her throat eased up enough for her to go back to sleep.

Patricia went to see a gastroenterologist, who started her on two different medications for acid reflux. Since she didn't want to take these medications indefinitely, she decided to get serious about diet and exercise. Over the next seven months, Patricia lost thirty pounds and was able to stop the medications. She was free of symptoms for the next three years. Recently, she regained fifteen pounds and has started having acid reflux symptoms again.

Natural Alternatives for Treating Acid Reflux

Beyond commonsense measures, there are several natural alternatives that can be used to alleviate acid reflux. People on the Mediterranean diet—fresh fruits and vegetables, fish, olive oil—have been reported to have less than half the incidence of acid reflux as those on a diet of red meat, fried food, sweets, and junk food. High-fiber foods—such as beans, fresh vegetables, and nuts—as well as digestive enzymes and probiotic supplements, available at health food stores and pharmacies, all help alleviate acid reflux.

Stress reduction techniques like listening to relaxation tapes, meditating, and exercising regularly can be helpful, since people exposed to chronic stress or having psychological problems are more likely to have symptoms of acid reflux. Some home remedies that can reduce acid reflux are aloe vera juice, licorice root, apple cider vinegar, ginger root, and slippery elm.

Acupuncture and Chinese herbs have been reported to be effective for acid reflux. One study evaluated the use of acupuncture for people who were taking PPIs but were still having troublesome symptoms. Participants were divided into two groups, half receiving a double dose of PPIs and the others adding acupuncture treatments to their current PPI dosage. After four weeks, those receiving acupuncture experienced a significant decrease in their symptoms, while those on the double dose of PPIs had no change.

My friend JT, a retired aerospace engineer, first noticed problems with heartburn after a trip to Japan with his wife. He had eaten spicier foods than usual and had sampled several varieties of strong Japanese liquor. When he returned to the United States, he visited his internist, who recommended *Zantac*, a common over-the counter medication. JT took one whenever he had heartburn, which helped right away, but it didn't stop him from having further episodes.

Concerned that this had become a chronic problem, he decided to see an acupuncturist recommended by a friend. After several treatments and also taking a daily Chinese herbal tablet, JT's heartburn became much less frequent and less severe. He still has an occasional flare-up after eating or drinking too much, but overall is much better since starting the Chinese herbs and acupuncture.

MEDICATIONS TO TREAT ACID REFLUX

If commonsense measures and natural alternatives are not reducing your symptoms to a tolerable level, then you should consider taking a medication. Several classes of drugs that might alleviate your symptoms are available over the counter or by prescription.

Antacids

If you have an occasional episode of heartburn after a big dinner out, a simple OTC antacid—*Pepto-Bismol*, *Maalox*, or *Tums*—might be enough to take away your symptoms. These preparations coat the lining of the stomach and neutralize stomach acid. Chronic use of these can cause problems such as diarrhea and constipation, however, and can affect the metabolism of calcium and magnesium in the body, dangerous for people with kidney problems.

H₂ Blockers

Up until the mid-1970s, antacids were the mainstay of treatment for heartburn and other symptoms of acid reflux. But at that time, H2 blockers—histamine H2-receptor antagonists—were developed to actually stop the secretion of acid in the stomach. These medications block the acid-making cells in the stomach lining from responding to histamine, reducing the amount of acid produced.

Cimetidine (*Tagamet*) became the first blockbuster drug in this category. Others, including *Pepcid* and *Zantac*, soon followed. These medications are available over the counter or in higher doses by prescription. Some of the side effects of H2 blockers include constipation, diarrhea, headache, dizziness, and skin rashes. The effectiveness of H2 blockers is mixed. While most people taking them report a reduction in their symptoms, one study found that only half of all users were completely free of symptoms.

PROTON PUMP INHIBITORS (PPIs)

Proton pump inhibitors, which were introduced in the late 1980s, have become the go-to for symptoms of acid reflux. They also are prescribed to prevent and treat ulcers that occur from taking anti-inflammatory drugs such as aspirin and ibuprofen, as well as for some uncommon conditions that cause damage to the esophagus.

PPIs are thought to be more effective than H2 blockers in reducing symptoms, although they sometimes take longer to start working. These drugs, which include *Nexium*, *Prevacid*, and *Prilosec*, reduce between 90 and 100 percent of stomach acid by inhibiting an enzyme—the "proton pump"—necessary for cells to produce acid. Studies have shown that all PPIs are equally effective in alleviating symptoms. Some are available OTC and others by prescription.

Your stomach produces acid for a reason—to help you digest food and absorb important nutrients. Taking a PPI in the short-term can help reduce your symptoms, but long-term use can be associated with a myriad of troubling health problems. PPIs were initially developed for short-term use of two weeks or less and FDA approvals were made with that in mind. Since then, the use of these blockbuster drugs has grown exponentially. Many patients now take them indefinitely, sometimes for relatively minor problems.

A study in Colorado of almost 6.6 million hospitalized patients who were taking PPIs reported that 73 percent did not need them. That's right—nearly five million people were taking PPIs needlessly, and this was just in Colorado. The patients taking PPIs also had an increased rate of *C. difficile*—a bacterial infection that causes diarrhea, abdominal cramping, and dehydration that can lead to kidney failure.

ADVERSE EFFECTS FROM PPIs

Common side effects that occur in up to 5 percent of PPI users include headaches, diarrhea, and abdominal pain. It is also becoming clear that long-term use can lead to many serious problems. Suppressing the production of stomach acid might alleviate your symptoms, but it comes with a definite downside.

Many essential nutrients—calcium, magnesium, iron, and vitamin B_{12}—require stomach acid in order to be absorbed by the body. Deficiencies of all of these can occur from taking PPIs, as well as from H2 blockers, since they also reduce stomach acid. As the list of medical problems associated with these medications grows, it is important for you to decide whether or not it is worthwhile to take them.

Vitamin B12 Deficiency

The *Journal of the American Medical Association* (*JAMA*) reported in 2013 that those taking PPIs for more than two years had nearly twice the incidence of vitamin B12 deficiency as nonusers. Vitamin B12 is not manufactured by the body. It is found in many animal-based foods such as meat, poultry, eggs, and dairy products, as well as in vitamin B12-enriched cereals, and in supplements. But if you have no stomach acid to absorb it, no matter how many of these things you eat or how many B12 supplements you take, it will not be incorporated into your body.

Vitamin B12 is necessary for the production of red blood cells. A deficiency of B12 can lead to a disease called pernicious anemia. Symptoms of this include fatigue, weakness, dizziness, shortness of breath, heart palpitations, numbness, tingling, depression, and memory loss.

Depression and Dementia

Vitamin B12 is also used in the synthesis of several important brain chemicals, such as serotonin and dopamine. There have been case reports of patients with severe depression and low vitamin

B12 levels who improved dramatically after receiving supplemental B12 therapy.

Evidence has now emerged that PPIs can increase the incidence of dementia, especially in the elderly. A German study of nearly 74,000 people aged seventy-five and older who did not initially have dementia reported that those taking a PPI had a 44 percent increased risk of developing dementia over the next several years.

The impact of such an increase in dementia could have profound implications. Even if only 3 percent of people in the United States over age seventy-five were taking PPIs, we could see 10,000 new cases of dementia each year. The effect of PPIs on dementia in younger people has not yet been studied.

Clostridium Difficile Infection

Clostridium difficile (*C. difficile*) is a diarrhea-causing bacterial infection that sometimes occurs after taking antibiotics, most often in the hospital. The connection between *C. difficile* and the use of stomach-acid suppressors, both PPIs and H2 blockers, was first reported in 2005. Researchers found that people who were taking PPIs were nearly three times more likely to have a *C. difficile* infection, while those on H2 blockers were twice as likely. Since stomach acids provide an important barrier to the invasion and growth of bacteria, researchers think that suppressing them leads to infection by *C. difficile*.

In February 2012, the FDA issued a safety announcement warning that the use of PPIs may be associated with an increased risk of *Clostridium difficile*–associated diarrhea. In a paper published that same year, the results of thirty different studies of more than 200,000 people were analyzed. Researchers reported that those on PPIs had twice the risk of having a *C. difficile* infection.

They noted that the growing epidemic of *C. difficile* infections had coincided with the exponential use of PPIs.

Changes in the *microbiome*—the mix of protective microorganisms living in your digestive tract—are another reason that PPIs increase the risk of gastrointestinal infections. People taking PPIs have fewer disease-fighting bacteria in their gut and more of the harmful ones. Some researchers believe that the effect PPIs have on reducing microbial diversity is greater than that of antibiotics or other commonly used drugs.

After heart surgery to replace her faulty aortic valve, Barbara's doctor put her on a PPI. He told her it was to prevent acid reflux, which might mimic heart problems, even though she had never had heartburn. Over the next two years, Barbara was hospitalized twice for food poisoning and dehydration. Her husband, who ate the same foods as she had, did not get sick either time. When Barbara was at the dentist's office, she read an article about PPIs reducing stomach acids, which can lead to gastrointestinal infections. She stopped taking her PPI and has had no further episodes of food poisoning, nor has she suffered from acid reflux.

Pneumonia

People taking PPIs have an increased risk of pneumonia, both within and outside the hospital. The reason for this is not entirely clear. A Dutch study reported that people who were taking PPIs were nearly two times as likely to develop pneumonia, compared to those who had used them in the past. The researchers also found that the results were dose dependent—people taking higher doses of PPIs were more likely to get pneumonia.

Another study reported that the risk of pneumonia is highest in the first week after starting a PPI and that people younger than age forty had more than twice the risk. The authors of a meta-analysis of thirty-one different studies concluded that both PPIs and H2 blockers increase the risk of pneumonia and urged doctors to use caution when prescribing them.

Bone Fractures

There is growing concern about the relationship between long-term use of PPIs and bone fractures. Since stomach acids are necessary for the absorption of calcium—vital for healthy bones—suppressing them could lead to thinning of the bones and subsequent fractures. Several studies have shown that older women taking PPIs have an increased risk of hip or spine fractures.

In the Nurses' Health Study, researchers followed nearly 80,000 postmenopausal women for fourteen years to track their use of PPIs and their incidence of hip fractures. After adjusting for other factors, such as obesity and certain drugs, they found that the risk of hip fracture in women who had regularly used PPIs for at least two years was 35 percent higher than the others.

The researchers then combined their results with those of ten other studies and found a similar result—a 25 to 35 percent increased risk of hip fractures in women taking PPIs. They cautioned that there was a "potential for a high burden of fractures attributable to PPIs across the population," due to the increasing use of them.

Studies also have reported that spine, wrist, and forearm fractures are associated with PPI use. Patients who take higher doses of PPIs have a greater risk of fractures, as well as those taking them for more than a year.

Chronic Kidney Disease

New evidence points to PPIs as the culprit in the rising incidence of chronic kidney disease (CKD). The number of people with CKD, many of them on twice-weekly dialysis treatments, has increased much faster than expected from known risk factors. At the same time, the use of PPIs has also increased. In a study of more than 10,000 participants followed for up to fourteen years, there was one and a half times the rate of CKD in PPI users compared to nonusers. During this same time, the use of PPIs in the population increased from 3.1 to more than 25 percent. The authors of the study wrote that up to 70 percent of these prescriptions were unnecessary and that 25 percent of long-term PPI users could discontinue therapy without developing symptoms.

Heart Disease

A 2015 study has raised alarm about a possible connection between PPIs and heart attacks. Researchers analyzed over sixteen million medical records from nearly three million patients and reported a 16 percent increased risk of heart attacks in people taking PPIs. A companion study in which the investigators followed PPI users over time was more disturbing. They found twice the risk of death from heart disease in those taking PPIs, while no increased risk was found in those taking H2 blockers. The authors speculated that this was due to reduced nitric oxide in blood vessel walls, a side effect of PPIs, which could lead to increased hardening of arteries and risk of blood clots.

These findings have met with some resistance within the medical community. It is possible that those who take PPIs are sicker in general and more prone to having heart attacks. In any event, the authors of the study cautioned that taking PPIs for more than two weeks is risky and suggested that other treatments for heartburn and acid reflux be considered for long-term use.

Stopping Your PPIs

It is not easy to stop taking PPIs after long-term use. This is due to a phenomenon known as *rebound hyperacidity*, in which stomach acid actually increases after stopping PPIs, causing symptoms of acid reflux to worsen. This was demonstrated in a fascinating 2009 study, in which people who did not have symptoms of acid reflux were randomly divided into two groups. One group received a placebo—a dummy sugar pill—for twelve weeks. The other one was given a PPI for eight weeks followed by four weeks of a placebo. During the last four weeks of the study, 44 percent of those who had taken the PPI for eight weeks had acid reflux symptoms compared to 15 percent of those who had taken the placebo for the entire time.

Stopping PPIs is difficult, but your stomach acid will eventually return to normal. Tapering off them gradually—switching to H2 blockers, and then progressing to simple antacids—and using commonsense methods and natural alternatives will help ease your discomfort.

Type of Acid Reflux Medication	Examples (Brand Name)	How They Work	Possible Side Effects
Simple antacid	Calcium carbonate (*Tums, Rolaids, Maalox*); Magnesium hydroxide (*Milk of Magnesia*); Aluminum hydroxide (*Mylanta, Di-Gel*); Bismuth subsalicylate (*Pepto-Bismol*)	Coat the lining of the stomach and neutralize stomach acid	Constipation, diarrhea, and imbalance of calcium and magnesium
Histamine H2-receptor antagonists (H2 blockers)	Cimetidine (*Tagamet*); Ranitidine (*Zantac*); Famotidine (*Pepcid*)	Block the acid-making cells in the stomach lining from responding to histamine	Constipation, diarrhea, headache, dizziness, and skin rashes; intestinal infections and pneumonia

Proton pump inhibitors (PPIs)	Omeprazole (*Prilosec*); Lansoprazole (*Prevacid*); Esomeprazole (*Nexium*)	Inhibit an enzyme—the proton pump—necessary for cells to produce acid	Headaches, diarrhea, and abdominal pain; vitamin B$_{12}$ deficiency, dementia, intestinal infections, pneumonia, bone fractures, chronic kidney disease, and heart disease

DO YOU REALLY NEED THAT ACID REFLUX PILL?

There are some conditions for which it is appropriate to take an H2 blocker or a PPI—short-term treatment of ulcers caused by a *Helicobacter pylori* infection, ulcers that occur from the long-term use of anti-inflammatory pain drugs such as aspirin and ibuprofen, and serious medical illnesses like ulcerative esophagitis, Barrett's esophagus, and Zollinger-Ellison syndrome. Sometimes, it is acceptable to use these medications temporarily to treat severe acid reflux not responsive to other treatments.

If you are among the vast majority of people with simple heartburn or acid reflux, taking these pills long-term is *not* indicated. Experts estimate that up to 70 percent of PPI prescriptions, the vast majority of those for acid reflux, are inappropriate. A prominent public health physician wrote that there are up to 80 million unnecessary prescriptions each year for PPIs, costing $9 billion worldwide. He advised that before prescribing these medications, doctors should weigh the seriousness of the patients' symptoms versus the seriousness of the possible adverse effects.

PPIs and other acid suppressors are very effective at relieving heartburn and other symptoms of acid reflux and can be used occasionally for severe discomfort after eating or drinking too much. Taking them long-term increases your risks of dementia, bone fractures, vitamin deficiencies, pneumonia, and intestinal infections. You are better off losing five to ten pounds, eating smaller meals, using natural alternatives, and taking simple antacids to alleviate your symptoms.

Do you really need that acid reflux pill? Most likely not.

Chapter 6

Depression

Depression is something many of us have experienced at one time or another. The breakup of a relationship, a job loss, the death of a family member—any of these can cause someone to become depressed. We would not be human if we did not have an emotional reaction to major life events. But is this normal reaction something that should cause a person to be medicated? When is depression significant enough for medication and what are the risks of taking an antidepressant?

Depression is widespread. In a government survey covering the years 2009–2012, 7.6 percent of people aged twelve and over in the United States reported moderate to severe symptoms of depression within the previous two weeks. The numbers were highest in women and people between the ages of forty and fifty-nine. An estimated 8 million doctor visits each year are for depression, half of which are to primary care doctors like family physicians and internists. The economic burden to the US economy from adults with depression has been estimated at more than $210 billion each year.

WHAT IS DEPRESSION?

Depression affects all aspects of a person's health. It can be acute, lasting only a few weeks, or it can become chronic, lasting two years or more. Its symptoms can be divided into three main categories:

- Emotional—sad, irritable, or depressed mood; loss of interest in usual activities; inability to experience pleasure; feelings of guilt or worthlessness; and thoughts of death or suicide
- Mental—inability to concentrate and difficulty making decisions
- Physical—fatigue, lack of energy, feeling either restless or slow, and changes in sleep, appetite, and activity levels

Causes of Depression

Depression is a complex process that is the result of the interplay between genetics, environmental stress, lifestyle, and biochemistry. Those with a family history of depression are more vulnerable to developing it, as are people with a history of physical, sexual, or emotional abuse. Stresses such as illness, divorce, job loss, grief, or even the birth of a child can lead to acute situational depression, which usually improves over time.

Economic hardship is also associated with depression. Depression is more common among the poor—more than 15 percent of people living below the federal poverty level had depression in the government survey compared to 6.2 percent of everyone else. People who are working and having trouble making ends meet often blame themselves for their problems.

Suicide rates increased by 24 percent in the fifteen years from 1999 through 2014, with the biggest jump starting after 2006, in tandem with the economic downturn. The largest increases occurred in those aged forty-five to sixty-four, with a 63 percent increase in suicide for women in that age group and a 43 percent increase for men. Suicides in this age group were most commonly related to job, financial, and legal problems.

People who are struggling with alcohol or substance abuse are more likely to experience depression as well as people dealing with a chronic illness. Sometimes depression is triggered by another medical condition, such as hypothyroidism, cancer, diabetes, or heart disease. Depression is also common in people experiencing chronic pain. In a survey of patients with chronic pain, more than three-fourths of them reported becoming depressed.

Certain medications can cause depression. From 8.4 to 11.6 percent of those taking newly prescribed opioid pain medication developed depression within the first thirty days, according to a study of more than 107,000 patients. Corticosteroid drugs such as prednisone, the antiviral drug interferon, and *Accutane* (isotretinoin), a drug used to treat acne, are all well known to cause depression. Other common drugs reported to cause depression include birth control pills, statin drugs, and antianxiety medications.

COMMON DRUGS THAT CAN CAUSE DEPRESSION

- Acne medications (*Accutane*)
- Seizure medications (*Zarontin*)
- Barbiturates (phenobarbital)
- Anxiety drugs (*Ativan, Valium, Xanax*)
- Beta blockers for blood pressure (*Lopressor, Tenormin*)

- Calcium channel blockers for blood pressure (*Cardizem, Procardia*)
- Opioid pain medications (*Vicodin, OxyContin,* morphine)
- Statins for high cholesterol (*Lipitor, Zocor, Crestor*)
- Antiviral drugs (interferon, *Zovirax*)
- Birth control pills

Types of Depression

Depression is classified by doctors as mild, moderate, or severe. This is often determined by answers to questions such as those on the Patient Health Questionnaire (PHQ–9), a nine-item screening instrument that asks about the frequency of symptoms of depression. An online version of this questionnaire can be found at patient.info/doctor/patient-health-questionnaire-phq-9. A person with a score of 5–9 is considered to have mild depression, 10–14 moderate, and 15 or more severe depression.

About 3 percent of people over age twelve in the United States have severe depression, also known as major depressive disorder (MDD). You are considered to have MDD if you have any five of the nine symptoms on the PHQ–9 *nearly every day* for more than two weeks. These are:

- depressed mood or irritable
- decreased interest or pleasure in most activities
- significant weight change (5 percent either lost or gained) or change in appetite
- change in sleep (either wakefulness or sleeping too much)

- change in activity level (either hyperactive or sluggish)
- fatigue or loss of energy
- feelings of guilt or worthlessness
- difficulty thinking, concentrating, or making decisions
- thoughts of suicide

Another type of depression that psychiatrists talk about is *dysthymia,* also called persistent depressive disorder. In this disorder, the symptoms are milder but are present for two years or more. For a diagnosis of dysthymia, a person needs two out of the following six symptoms for at least two years: poor appetite or overeating, insomnia or sleeping too much, low energy or fatigue, low self-esteem, poor concentration or difficulty making decisions, and feelings of hopelessness. Many people experience two or more of these symptoms at one time or another, but it is rare to have them for such an extended period.

MANAGING DEPRESSION WITHOUT DRUGS

There are many ways to manage depression without drugs. A comprehensive US government review reported that nonpharmacological treatments for major depression had similar benefits to medication with a lower risk of adverse events. Psychotherapy, exercise, acupuncture, and St. John's wort were some of the interventions evaluated in this review. Healthy diets, omega-3 fatty acids, nutritional supplements, sunlight, meditation, biofeedback, and homeopathy are additional options that can help people with depression.

Psychotherapy

The American College of Physicians recommends that cognitive behavioral therapy (CBT) be strongly considered as the first-line treatment for major depression. This came after a review of studies from 1990 through 2015 reported that CBT was just as effective as antidepressant medications, without the dangers of serious side effects. These studies also showed that patients taking medication were more likely to discontinue treatment and that combining CBT with drug therapy was more effective than drug therapy alone. In the large Sequenced Treatment Alternatives to Relieve Depression (STAR*D) study, cognitive therapy was as effective as switching to a different antidepressant for those who did not improve after twelve weeks of initial drug therapy.

Cognitive behavioral therapy is a short-term therapy in which the connection between a person's thoughts and behaviors is explored. The goal is to change patterns of negative thoughts or behaviors that affect how a person feels. CBT is not always covered by insurance and it can be hard to find a practitioner in a local area. But given the headaches, insomnia, constipation, diarrhea, sexual dysfunction, dizziness, and drowsiness that are associated with drug therapy, it is an option that someone should seriously consider.

Other forms of psychotherapy, including interpersonal and psychodynamic therapies, have also been reported to be as effective as drug therapy. But, like with CBT, it can be difficult to find a therapist that is covered by insurance. Few psychiatrists engage in psychotherapy these days, generally limiting their practices to medication management. A psychiatrist can earn up to $150 for three fifteen-minute medication visits compared with $90 for a forty-five-minute talk therapy session.

Exercise

There is no doubt that exercise helps to manage depression. For one thing, exercise stimulates the production of endorphins and other chemicals in the brain that affect mood, sometimes creating a temporary state of euphoria, also known as the "runner's high." Exercise also enhances self-esteem, reduces stress, and improves sleep. It can be done on your own, without a prescription.

An analysis of thirty-seven studies of exercise and depression concluded that exercise improves symptoms of depression as much as psychological or pharmacological therapies. In one study, adults aged twenty to forty-five years old who exercised three to five times per week for thirty minutes reduced their symptoms of depression by almost 50 percent after twelve weeks.

There is evidence that exercise might give more long-lasting relief from depression than medication. In a study of 156 adults, 60 to 70 percent of participants in all three treatment groups (exercise alone, medication alone, combined exercise and medication) no longer had major depression after sixteen weeks. After ten months, those in the exercise alone group had lower rates of relapse, especially those who continued to exercise on their own.

Aerobic exercise is most often recommended for depression, but strength training is also important. It can be hard for someone who is depressed to have the motivation to start exercising. But even a walk around the block once a day is a good start. After a while, the benefits of exercise should outweigh the feelings of lassitude. Before undertaking an exercise program, make sure to consult your doctor.

Diet and Nutritional Supplements

Your diet can have a profound effect on your chances of having depression. Studies have shown that those who have high intakes of fruit, vegetables, fish, and whole grains have less risk of depression. There is also evidence that people who are depressed have low blood levels of folic acid, found in fruits and leafy green vegetables, and vitamin B12, which comes from meat and dairy products.

In a recent study of nearly 70,000 postmenopausal women, researchers reported that eating refined carbohydrates and added sugars increased the risk of depression, while women who ate more fiber, fruits, and vegetables had lower rates of depression. Other studies have shown that the Mediterranean diet decreased the risk of becoming depressed while diets high in processed foods were associated with increased odds of developing depression.

There is good evidence that omega-3 fatty acids, found in fish oil, are effective in treating depression. An analysis of nineteen studies comparing omega-3s with placebos reported that they were effective for patients with major depressive disorder as well as those with less severe symptoms of depression. The best sources of omega-3 fatty acids are fatty fish such as mackerel, salmon, and herring. Cod liver oil and other fish oil supplements are available for those who do not regularly eat fish. Non-fish sources of omega-3 fatty acids include flaxseed oil, chia seeds, walnuts, and soybeans.

Nutritional supplements are also used by some doctors to treat depression. Tryptophan is an amino acid that is important in the synthesis of serotonin, a neurotransmitter in the brain. It is given in the form of 5-hydroxytryptophan (5-HTP) and has been found to be better than placebo in treating depression in a few studies. Side effects of 5-HTP include dizziness, nausea, and diarrhea.

Another supplement that is used to treat depression is SAMe, or S-adenosylmethionine, which is necessary for the production of serotonin, norepinephrine, and dopamine—brain chemicals thought to be associated with mood. SAMe treatment was as effective as antidepressants and better than placebo in treating patients with major depression, according to a 2010 meta-analysis. Vitamin C also has been reported to help depressed patients in several studies.

Sunlight

Sunlight is important in fighting depression in two ways. The first is the therapeutic effect of light itself. Studies show that exposure to light improves seasonal affective disorder (SAD), which occurs in winter months from lack of sunlight. The reason light helps depression is not well understood, but scientists believe it has something to do with reestablishing normal circadian rhythms. The effect of light on major depression, until recently, has not been known.

A placebo-controlled study comparing light therapy (a fluorescent white-light box for thirty minutes in the morning), an SSRI antidepressant, and a combination of the two was carried out in patients with moderate-to-severe MDD. After eight weeks, light therapy was more effective than the antidepressant and significantly better than the placebo. Those receiving the combination of light therapy and antidepressant improved the most.

The other benefit of sunlight comes from vitamin D. In a study of 185 young women in the Pacific Northwest, those who had low vitamin D levels were more likely to have clinically significant symptoms of depression. This was after researchers controlled for other factors that could contribute to depression, such as diet, exercise, and time spent outdoors. Two recent meta-analyses, which summarized the findings from several different studies, reported that supplementation with vitamin D was effective in treating people with clinically significant depression. Several high-quality studies showed that vitamin D had an effect that was comparable to that of antidepressant medication.

For more specifics on vitamin D and supplementation, see the osteoporosis chapter.

St. John's Wort

The herb St. John's wort—scientific name *Hypericum perforatum*—has a long history of use for depression, anxiety, and insomnia, especially in Europe. It has a yellow star-shaped flower and often grows wild in the United States. A review of twenty-nine different studies, carried out by the internationally recognized Cochrane Collaboration, reported that St. John's wort was better than placebo in treating patients with major depression and was just as effective as a standard antidepressant, with fewer side effects. It is thought to act by increasing the level of serotonin, a neurotransmitter that affects mood, in the brain.

St. John's wort is available over the counter in liquid or pill form and the dried herb can be used to make a tea. A typical dose is 300 milligrams three times a day. Taking St. John's wort with other medications that also affect serotonin, including antidepressants, increases the chance of developing serotonin syndrome, a rare but potentially fatal occurrence (see chapter 1). Another thing to be aware of with St. John's wort is that it can decrease the blood levels of several common medications, including warfarin, digoxin (for heart failure), theophylline (for asthma), amitriptyline (for depression), cholesterol-lowering agents, and the erectile dysfunction drug *Viagra*.

Acupuncture and Homeopathy

Acupuncture has been used for hundreds of years in China to treat depression but had not been evaluated by modern research methods until recently. A meta-analysis of twenty high-quality studies reported that acupuncture treatment is comparable to antidepressants in alleviating symptoms of depression in patients with major depressive disorder. That same analysis reported that, as you might expect, the incidence of adverse effects was significantly lower with acupuncture compared to antidepressants.

Other studies have shown that when acupuncture is added to antidepressants, the results are better than those for antidepressants alone. Seven hundred and fifty-five patients who were being treated for depression were randomized to add acupuncture or counseling to what they were taking or to continue their usual treatment. Two-thirds of them were taking antidepressants. After three months, those receiving acupuncture treatment or counseling had significantly lower scores on the PHQ-9 depression test than the others.

Homeopathy, which is widely used in Europe, Latin America, and India, is another alternative that can be used to treat depression. Patients take small doses of natural substances to stimulate the body's self-healing ability. In a recent study, 133 middle-aged Mexican women with moderate-to-severe depression were randomized to receive either individualized homeopathic treatment, an antidepressant, or a placebo. After six weeks, the homeopathic group showed a statistically significant decrease in symptoms compared to placebo, with results that were equivalent to the group receiving the antidepressant. These results are similar to those of a previous study that found that individualized homeopathic treatment was as effective as fluoxetine (*Prozac*) in the treatment of people with moderate or severe depression. Homeopathy is practiced by specially trained naturopathic physicians, medical doctors, nurse practitioners, and other health providers.

Mindfulness Meditation

Mindfulness meditation has been combined with cognitive therapy to provide a technique known as mindfulness-based cognitive therapy (MBCT). Patients learn the technique of sitting quietly with their eyes closed and concentrating on the rhythm of their breathing for twenty to thirty minutes each day. The purpose is to detach from negative thought patterns and break the downward spiral into depression.

MBCT shows great promise, especially in preventing relapses in those with chronic depression. Patients who have had several bouts of depression sometimes do not like taking antidepressants long-term and discontinue them, leading to recurrence of their symptoms. In a study comparing MBCT with maintenance antidepressants in patients with recurrent bouts of depression, both therapies were equally effective in preventing relapses or recurrences over a two-year period. For patients with a history of childhood abuse, MBCT was better than antidepressants.

The results of an analysis that combined data from nine similar studies were even more interesting. Researchers reported that patients using MBCT had a significantly lower risk of recurring depression than those taking antidepressants, especially those who were suffering from more severe depression at the beginning of treatment. In the United Kingdom, the National Institute for Health and Care Excellence (NICE) has recommended MBCT as a treatment for depression since 2004.

My cousin Richard, a thirty-seven-year-old database manager, suffered a sprained ankle that wouldn't heal. Concerned that the pain would become chronic, he became depressed and anxious. Poor appetite, disturbed sleep, and lack of energy soon followed. After several months, his primary care doctor referred him to a psychiatrist for antidepressant medication.

The side effects of the medication made Richard feel terrible. He had continuous nausea with dryness and a bad taste in his mouth. He gained twenty pounds and his fatigue became worse. He was switched to a different medication with no improvement. Finally, his sister recommended that he try mindfulness meditation.

Richard tapered off the antidepressant and enrolled in a six-week meditation class. He started meditating daily. After two months, the difference was striking. His sleep improved, he lost fifteen pounds, and his outlook improved considerably. He told me that mindfulness meditation helped him to understand the connection between his body and his emotions and how to control them.

Yoga, Massage, and Biofeedback

Since depression is related to stress, it makes sense that techniques that are meant to reduce stress would be helpful in managing depression. Yoga has been found to be useful in a wide range of mental health disorders, including depression. Massage therapy helps alleviate symptoms of depression, according to a meta-analysis of seventeen randomized, controlled studies. Studies of biofeedback have also demonstrated significant improvements in depression scores after several sessions.

NONDRUG TREATMENTS FOR DEPRESSION

- Psychotherapy—cognitive behavioral, interpersonal, psychodynamic, and others
- Exercise—three to five times weekly for thirty minutes
- Diet—high in fresh fruits and vegetables, fiber, and fish (or other omega-3 fatty acid sources)
- Alternative therapies—acupuncture, St. John's wort, homeopathy
- Sun exposure—or light therapy and vitamin D supplementation
- Mindfulness meditation
- Yoga, massage, and biofeedback

ANTIDEPRESSANT MEDICATION

In national surveys, the number of people in the United States who reported taking an antidepressant in the previous thirty days grew from 1.8 percent in the period of 1988 to 1994 to nearly 9 percent from 2007 to 2010. A Mayo Clinic survey found that more than 12 percent of people were taking an antidepressant, including *26 percent of women between the ages of fifty and sixty-four*. According to these surveys, more people took antidepressants (9 to 12 percent) than were reported to have depression (7.6 percent). This is disturbing, especially given the evidence that many nondrug therapies are as effective as taking medication.

One reason that so many people take antidepressants is that pharmaceutical companies promote them vigorously, not only to consumers, but also to medical providers for "off-label" uses. This means that doctors are encouraged, often at lavish dinners and all-expenses-paid trips, to prescribe them for medical conditions not included in their FDA approval. A recent Canadian study reported that only 55.2 percent of prescriptions for antidepressants by primary care providers were for depression. The rest were prescribed for conditions such as anxiety, insomnia, and pain.

The practice of encouraging off-label use has cost the drug companies *billions* of dollars in fines, which are generally seen as part of the cost of doing business. For example, GlaxoSmith-Kline was fined $3 billion for promoting the antidepressant *Paxil* to children and *Wellbutrin*, another antidepressant, to adults for weight gain, sexual dysfunction, ADHD, and bulimia. Even with this huge fine, the company still made a considerable profit, with $17.5 billion in sales of these two drugs during the years covered by the settlement.

How Effective Are Antidepressant Medications?

There is no class of drugs for which there is so little evidence of effectiveness as antidepressants, especially for people with mild to moderate depression. In a meta-analysis of data from six different studies, the benefit of antidepressant medication in patients with mild or moderate symptoms was found to be minimal to nonexistent compared to placebo. Researchers say that this is because up to 40 percent of people will improve from taking a placebo. Antidepressants would have to cause improvement in *more* than 40 percent of people in these studies to be considered better than a placebo. This begs the question—if a placebo can help 40 percent of people, why not give them that instead of an antidepressant? In fact, there is recent evidence that the placebo response activates natural opioids in the body, leading to antidepressive effects.

There is no doubt that some people are helped by antidepressants. In the meta-analysis of six different studies, antidepressants were superior to placebo only in patients with very severe depression. An analysis by the Cochrane Collaboration reported that for every seven to eight people treated with selective serotonin reuptake inhibitors (SSRIs), only one person would benefit. The effect of antidepressants is small and becomes clinically significant only in people who are the most severely depressed, according to another meta-analysis. Researchers concluded that "there is little reason to prescribe new-generation antidepressant medications to any but the most severely depressed patients unless alternative treatments have been ineffective."

Other studies have reported that less than half of those with major depression receive benefits after taking antidepressants for a full year. In the government-sponsored STAR*D study of almost 3,000 people with moderate or severe depression, only one-third of participants became symptom-free after taking an antidepressant for up to twelve weeks. For those still depressed, a second, third, or fourth medicine was added over the course of a year. By the end of that time, 30 percent of patients still had MDD and nearly 50 percent of them had dropped out, presumably from adverse side effects.

There is also evidence that negative studies of antidepressants are published in medical journals much less frequently than positive ones. In the analysis of seventy-four studies registered with the FDA that was reported in chapter 2, only 51 percent showed positive results. However, because more of them were published, it appeared as though 94 percent of these trials were positive.

The Biochemical Theory of Depression

There is a widely-held belief that depression is due to a "biochemical imbalance" in the brain—specifically, that people who are depressed have low levels of certain brain chemicals, such as serotonin, norepinephrine, and dopamine. Advertising by pharmaceutical companies has largely revolved around the claim that antidepressants can correct this chemical imbalance, leading to blockbuster drugs such as *Zoloft*, *Prozac*, *Paxil*, *Effexor*, and *Cymbalta*.

While biochemical abnormalities might be a factor in depression for some people, there are other things that can trigger it as well. Focusing solely on the pharmaceutical approach not only fails to address other issues, but creates the false impression that people are passive victims, powerless to do anything on their own to feel better. As we've seen already, there are many nondrug approaches to treating depression.

The majority of drugs prescribed for depression are given to increase serotonin levels in the brain. However, there is no conclusive evidence that low serotonin in the brain is associated with depression since it is impossible to measure this in a living person. Eighty percent of serotonin is found in the gastrointestinal system, where it regulates smooth muscle contraction. It is also found in blood platelets, where it contributes to clotting, as well as in the brain.

Experiments to induce depression by depleting serotonin have not produced consistent results, suggesting that some people may be more susceptible to low serotonin than others. Low blood levels of serotonin have been found in depressed people but it isn't known if these are related to the levels in the brain, since serotonin cannot cross the barrier between the bloodstream and the brain. Also unknown is whether low serotonin levels are the *cause* of depression or a *result* of it—the chicken-and-the-egg conundrum.

One argument given to justify the serotonin hypothesis is that drugs that elevate serotonin have been shown to help some people with depression. Using this same reasoning, one might conclude that headaches are due to an aspirin deficiency. One psychiatry professor has gone so far as to declare that the concept that depression is the result of low serotonin levels is a myth, perpetuated by clever marketing that has turned depression into a biochemical entity rather than what some might consider to be a "moral weakness."

Tricyclic Antidepressants

Tricyclic antidepressants (TCAs) such as imipramine (*Tofranil*) and amitriptyline (*Elavil*) were first discovered in the 1950s and were the primary drugs used to treat depression until the selective serotonin reuptake inhibitors (SSRIs) came onto the market in the late 1980s. TCAs block the reuptake of the neurotransmitters serotonin and norepinephrine by nerve cells, resulting in higher levels of these chemicals in the brain. They are also potent anticholinergics (see chapter 1) and are sometimes still used today. They fell out of favor because their side effects seemed to be greater than those of the SSRIs. Another factor could be because their patents expired and the newer SSRIs became more profitable.

Side Effects of Tricyclic Antidepressants

The side effects of TCAs include dry mouth, constipation, dizziness, drowsiness, weight gain, and sexual dysfunction. Although these symptoms are worrisome, a more serious concern is that TCAs have been linked to an increased risk of dementia, due to their anticholinergic properties. They also have been linked to an increase in suicidal thoughts and behavior, especially at the beginning of treatment. A British study of nearly 160,000 patients taking tricyclic or SSRI antidepressants revealed that fatal suicides were thirty-eight times more likely to occur during the first ten days of treatment compared to ninety days later.

Monoamine Oxidase Inhibitors

Monoamine oxidase inhibitors (MAOIs), another class of antidepressants, elevate the levels of three brain chemicals associated with mood—norepinephrine, serotonin, and dopamine. They are not often used because of serious interactions with other drugs, including tricyclic and SSRI antidepressants, asthma medications, and antihistamine/decongestants. They also should not be taken with foods containing high levels of the amino acid tyrosine, which regulates blood pressure. Such foods include aged cheeses, cured or smoked meats, beer, red wine, soy products, sauerkraut, brewer's yeast, and other fermented foods. MAOIs are mostly used for people who do not benefit from other types of antidepressants. Examples of MAOIs are phenelzine (*Nardil*), isocarboxazid (*Marplan*), and tranylcypromine (*Parnate*).

Side Effects of MAOIs

Side effects of MAOIs include dry mouth, nausea, headache, insomnia, diarrhea or constipation, and dizziness or light-headedness. Eating foods containing tyrosine can cause a dangerous spike in blood pressure. There is also a risk of the potentially fatal serotonin syndrome when taken with other serotonin-enhancing drugs or herbs such as migraine and pain medications, certain antibiotics, St. John's wort, and other classes of antidepressants (see chapter 1).

SSRIs and SNRIs

Selective serotonin reuptake inhibitors (SSRIs) and serotonin and norepinephrine reuptake inhibitors (SNRIs) are collectively referred to as "second-generation" antidepressants because they came on the market later than the TCAs or MAOIs. The most frequently used are the SSRIs. Medications in this class include fluoxetine (*Prozac*), paroxetine (*Paxil*), sertraline (*Zoloft*), and many others. They inhibit the reuptake of the neurotransmitter serotonin, increasing the amount of it available in the brain.

Serotonin and norepinephrine reuptake inhibitors (SNRIs) increase the amount of another brain chemical, norepinephrine, in addition to serotonin. Venlafaxine (*Effexor*) and duloxetine (*Cymbalta*) are examples of SNRIs. They are sometimes prescribed for anxiety and pain, as well as for depression. Studies have not shown any significant differences between SSRIs and SNRIs in treating depression, although the SNRIs are reported to be better tolerated in some patients. SNRIs are associated with more severe withdrawal symptoms and should not be stopped all at once.

Side Effects of SSRIs and SNRIs

Sixteen to 29 percent of people who start therapy with antidepressants stop taking them within three months. The discontinuation rate is as much as 36 percent in patients aged fifty-five and older. These medications can cause a host of unpleasant side effects, including gastrointestinal symptoms such as nausea, diarrhea, and constipation as well as dry mouth, insomnia, headaches, fatigue, and weight gain. Also problematic are the sexual side effects—decreased desire, poor erections, and difficulty reaching orgasm. There are several more serious issues, including, like the MAOIs, the risk of the dangerous serotonin syndrome when taken with certain other drugs.

Suicidal, Aggressive, and Violent Behavior

The most disturbing adverse effects of serotonin-inhibiting antidepressants are those that affect behavior. Not only are suicidal thoughts increased at the beginning of therapy with these medications, but suicide attempts occur more frequently as well. In an exhaustive analysis of 702 trials including almost 88,000 people with depression, there were more than twice as many suicide attempts in those taking SSRIs compared to those given placebos or therapies other than tricyclic antidepressants.

The greatest concerns about suicide and SSRIs are in young people. In 2007, the FDA ordered a black box warning that read, "Antidepressants increased the risk compared to placebo of suicidal thinking and behavior (suicidality) in children, adolescents, and young adults (ages eighteen to twenty-four) in short-term studies of major depressive disorder (MDD) and other psychiatric disorders." This warning, which is still in effect, alerted parents and caregivers to report any unusual changes in behavior, deepening depression, or thoughts of suicide to the patient's health-care provider. Subsequent studies have shown that there is a 58 percent increased risk of suicidal thoughts and behavior in children and adolescents taking antidepressants and that those taking higher doses have a greater risk of harming themselves.

According to a review of data in Europe, there is more than twice the risk of suicidal and aggressive behavior in children and adolescents taking SSRI and SNRI antidepressants. The authors also reported that, due to lack of access to individual case reports from drug companies, these results were likely an underestimate of actual harms. Even more alarming, a review of adverse drug events from the FDA database revealed that SSRI and SNRI antidepressants were more than eight times as likely to be associated with violent behavior than other drugs assessed.

Antidepressant-induced violent behavior has been used as a legal defense in several cases involving homicide, including that of Andrea Yates, the young mother who drowned her five children in a bathtub while taking *Effexor*, a SNRI, in 2001. A 2015 Swedish study found a 43 percent increased rate of convictions for violent crimes in those aged fifteen to twenty-four who were taking SSRIs. In a laboratory experiment, repeated doses of a common antidepressant (*Prozac*) stimulated parts of the brain associated with violent behavior in rats.

Strokes and Upper GI Bleeding

There is an increased risk of bleeding problems with second-generation antidepressants. This is due to a lower concentration of serotonin in blood platelets, which interferes with the ability to clot. People taking these medications have more than one and a half times the risk of developing upper gastrointestinal bleeding, especially when combined with nonsteroidal anti-inflammatory drugs such as aspirin and ibuprofen.

The use of serotonin-enhancing antidepressants has also been associated with strokes. A recent meta-analysis reported a 40 percent increase in strokes in those using them. People taking these antidepressants are also more than twice as likely to experience microbleeds, small unnoticed strokes in the brain that have been associated with mental impairment and Alzheimer's disease.

Low Blood Sodium, Diabetes, Falls, and Overall Mortality

A potentially life-threatening problem for those taking SSRIs is hyponatremia, or an abnormally low level of sodium in the blood. This is due to the effect they have on water elimination in the kidneys. Older people and those taking thiazide diuretics, which also affect the body's water balance, are particularly at risk for this complication. Symptoms include nausea and vomiting, headache, fatigue, muscle spasms, seizures, and eventually coma, if not treated appropriately. Other classes of antidepressants have also been found to cause hyponatremia, including SNRIs and tricyclics.

People who are taking antidepressants of all kinds are more at risk of developing type 2 diabetes. Part of this is due to the link between depression—often accompanied by obesity and poor lifestyle choices—and diabetes. But a study of nearly 36,000 African American women followed for twelve years reported that those taking antidepressants were 26 percent more likely to develop diabetes, independent of their lifestyle factors and body weight.

Fractures and falls have also been found to be more common in people taking antidepressants, with the highest risks in those taking SSRIs. In an analysis of more than 60,000 patients aged sixty-five and over diagnosed with depression, the risk of falls was 66 percent higher and the risk of death from any cause was 54 percent higher in those taking SSRIs than in those not taking medication.

Antidepressants During Pregnancy

It is estimated that 6 to 10 percent of pregnant women take antidepressants. This is alarming, given the evidence that birth defects and autism are more common in the children of women who take them. While some of these linkages are controversial, it is safer for pregnant women to have an abundance of caution and use psychotherapy or other nonpharmacologic approaches instead of medications to treat depression.

Birth Defects

The most common birth defects associated with antidepressants are holes in the chambers of the heart. Other birth defects include cleft palate and anencephaly—a fatal condition that occurs when the brain and parts of the skull don't develop.

Antidepressants have been linked with another very serious birth defect called persistent pulmonary hypertension of the newborn (PPHN). This condition affects the heart and lungs and makes it difficult for the baby to breathe. Although rare, it can lead to brain damage and even death. In 2006, the FDA issued a warning that SSRIs may be associated with this syndrome but in 2011 said that the connection was not so clear. Since then, it has been estimated that one case of PPHN is likely to occur for every 286 to 351 women taking SSRIs in late pregnancy.

Autism

Studies suggest that there may be a connection between the epidemic of autism spectrum disorder (ASD) and antidepressants. In a study published in 2016, researchers analyzed data from more than 145,000 children born in Quebec during a two-year period who were followed for more than six years. Mothers who had taken SSRIs during the last six months of pregnancy were more than twice as likely to have a child with ASD. Researchers speculated that serotonin might hinder brain development, which occurs during this period of time. Another study, published in 2014, reported that boys whose mothers took SSRIs during pregnancy were nearly three times as likely to have ASD, as well as other developmental delays. This research provides another reason that pregnant women should avoid antidepressants.

Other Antidepressant Medications

There are several other antidepressants that are less commonly used. Most of them inhibit various combinations of brain chemicals thought to affect mood. These medications are all relatively new so the long-term side effects are unknown. They include:

- Bupropion (*Wellbutrin*), which affects norepinephrine and dopamine. Reports show less weight gain and sexual side effects than with other antidepressants. Side effects include headache, insomnia, anxiety, and upset stomach.
- Mirtazapine (*Remeron*), which affects norepinephrine and serotonin. Side effects include sleepiness, weight gain, dizziness, and elevated triglycerides in the blood.
- Trazodone (*Oleptro*), a serotonin antagonist and reuptake inhibitor (SARI) that is also used to treat insomnia. Side effects include dizziness, drowsiness, blurred vision, vomiting, headache, and nausea. It can cause serotonin syndrome when used with MAOIs or other antidepressants.

Withdrawal from Antidepressants

It is not easy to stop taking antidepressants. While they are not considered addictive, withdrawal symptoms occur in about 20 percent of people taking them for at least six weeks when antidepressants are stopped abruptly. These symptoms usually appear within a few days of stopping the drug and can last for several weeks or even months. Sometimes they are mistaken for a relapse of depression or a new illness and new drugs are prescribed.

In a review of fifteen studies, symptoms such as anxiety, depression, flulike symptoms, muscle spasms, tremors, insomnia, headaches, and fatigue were reported with antidepressant withdrawal. More serious ones were confusion, panic attacks, bizarre dreams, suicidal thoughts, and hallucinations. SNRIs such as *Effexor* and *Cymbalta*, which affect both serotonin and norepinephrine, are the most likely to cause withdrawal symptoms but they can occur from SSRIs as well. Symptoms are worse in patients who stop their medications suddenly, but they also occur in those who taper off gradually. If you decide to stop taking an antidepressant, make sure you do so under the supervision of your doctor.

Type of Antidepressant	Examples (Brand Name)	How They Work	Possible Side Effects
Tricyclic (TCAs)	Imipramine (*Tofranil*); Amitriptyline (*Elavil*)	Elevate the levels of serotonin and norepinephrine in the brain	Dry mouth, constipation, dizziness, drowsiness, weight gain, and sexual dysfunction; dementia
Monoamine oxidase inhibitors (MAOIs)	Phenelzine (*Nardil*); Isocarboxazid (*Marplan*); Tranylcypromine (*Parnate*)	Elevate levels of norepinephrine, serotonin, and dopamine in the brain	Dry mouth, nausea, headache, insomnia, diarrhea or constipation, dizziness; dangerous high blood pressure when taken with certain foods; risk of serotonin syndrome

Selective serotonin reuptake inhibitors (SSRIs)	Fluoxetine (*Prozac*); Paroxetine (*Paxil*); Sertraline (*Zoloft*); Citalopram (*Celexa*); Escitalopram (*Lexapro*)	Elevate levels of serotonin in the brain	Dry mouth, nausea, diarrhea, constipation, insomnia, head-aches, fatigue, and weight gain; sexual dysfunc-tion. Risk of sero-tonin syndrome. Suicidal and violent behavior, strokes, upper GI bleeding, diabetes, falls, increased death rates, birth defects, and autism
Serotonin and norepi-nephrine reuptake inhibitors (SNRIs)	Venlafaxine (*Effexor*); Duloxetine (*Cymbalta*); Desvenlafax-ine (*Pristiq*)	Elevate levels of serotonin and norepinephrine in the brain	Same as SSRIs except withdrawal syndrome more severe
Others	Bupropion (*Wellbutrin*)	Elevates norepi-nephrine and dopamine	Headache, insom-nia, anxiety, and upset stomach; less weight gain and sexual side effects

| Others (cont.) | Mirtazapine (*Remeron*) | Elevates serotonin and norepinephrine | Sleepiness, weight gain, dizziness, and elevated triglycerides in the blood |
| | Trazodone (*Oleptro*) | Serotonin antagonist and reuptake inhibitor | Dizziness, drowsiness, blurred vision, vomiting, headache, and nausea |

DO YOU REALLY NEED THAT ANTIDEPRESSANT PILL?

In deciding whether or not to take an antidepressant, it is important to balance the potential benefits with the potential harms. For the vast majority of people with depression, studies have repeatedly shown that nondrug therapies—psychotherapy, exercise, acupuncture, and others—are equally effective if not more so than antidepressants. Even in people with severe depression, less than half of them will be helped by an antidepressant and it may take several tries over weeks or months to find the right one.

On the other hand, antidepressants have numerous potential harms. Suicide, violent behavior, bleeding disorders, diabetes, and an increased risk of birth defects and autism in the unborn child have all been associated with them. Stopping an antidepressant is often difficult and can cause symptoms worse than those being treated.

It takes more effort to exercise, change your diet, meditate, or visit a behavioral therapist or acupuncturist than it does to take a pill. You might be one of those lucky one-out-of-seven people for whom antidepressants are effective and you might not suffer any ill effects. But if you want to play it safe, you would be wise to investigate nondrug therapies first. In the end, it's up to you to decide whether or not you *really* need that pill.

Chapter 7

Chronic Pain: Back, Neck, and Osteoarthritic

Chronic pain affects at least 100 million Americans, more people than diabetes, heart disease, and cancer combined. The cost to the US economy is approximately $600 billion each year, half of which is spent on health-care costs, the other half due to lost productivity of workers. Worldwide, 1.5 billion people suffer from chronic pain.

Low back pain is the most common type of chronic pain. In a 2014 survey, more than 28 percent of US adults reported having low back pain within the previous three months. In people aged sixty-five and above, one-third reported having had it. Fortunately, most back pain goes away within a few weeks and does not require an X-ray or prescription medication. But in 10 to 15 percent of people, back pain becomes chronic, lasting more than three months. Many people report more than one type of chronic pain. Fifteen percent of people report they have had neck pain, 19.5 percent shoulder pain, 9 percent knee pain, 7.6 percent finger pain, and 7 percent hip pain.

The epidemic of prescription drug abuse in the United States stems primarily from opioid pain relievers. You might remember that my mother-in-law, Arlyn, ended up in the hospital with kidney failure after taking too much morphine (an opioid) for low back pain. She was relatively lucky. In 2016, there were more than 64,000 deaths from opiate overdoses. Many of these people were taking legally prescribed medications for chronic pain. Others became addicted while taking them and continued taking them illegally when their prescriptions ran out.

I remember a period in the early 2000s when doctors were encouraged to be lenient in prescribing opiates. The prevailing thought was that it was wrong to let people suffer from pain when it could be alleviated with these drugs, which were relatively inexpensive. That philosophy has backfired and we now have an epidemic of drug abuse that is out of control. The US government is now calling for stricter rules in opioid prescribing as doctors scramble to find alternatives for treating patients with chronic pain.

BACK PAIN

Eighty percent of adults suffer from back pain at some time in their lives. It is the leading cause of disability and missed work worldwide. It can be caused by muscle strains from a sudden injury or from the repeated stress of heavy lifting. Damage or degeneration of the vertebral disks—the soft, spongy material between the bones of the spine—is another cause. Ruptured or bulging disks can press against the nerves leaving the spinal column, causing back pain.

In older people, back pain can result from osteoarthritis of the spine causing inflammation or spinal stenosis—a narrowing of the disk openings. Osteoporosis also can cause the spinal bones to become brittle and collapse, leading to compression fractures. Though rare, a tumor in the spinal column can cause back pain, so be sure to tell your doctor if you have persistent pain.

There are several things you can do to reduce your risk of back pain. Bend your knees when lifting something heavy to help take the strain off your back. Lose weight and exercise—extra pounds put added strain on your back and lack of exercise can cause your back muscles to become weak. Even smoking has been linked to an increase in back pain, although the specific reason for this is unclear.

Managing Back Pain without Drugs

There are many strategies for managing back pain without drugs. The guidelines of two prominent physician groups recommend that patients with new-onset low back pain remain active and use self-care measures, such as exercise, ice, heat, and over-the-counter (OTC) pain medications. They also recommend non-pharmacologic treatments, such as exercise therapy, acupuncture, massage therapy, spinal manipulation, yoga, and cognitive behavioral therapy, all of which have been shown to be effective.

These guidelines for new-onsest pain also recommend against initial X-rays or other imaging studies, as well as prescription pain relievers. Unfortunately, some doctors do not follow this advice. A survey of general practice physicians reported that more than 25 percent of them referred patients with new low back pain for magnetic resonance imaging (MRI) testing and nearly 20 percent prescribed opioid pain medications before recommending more conservative approaches.

Physical Therapy

Physical therapy is practiced by trained professionals who use a variety of treatments—massage, spinal manipulation, heat or ice treatments, and electrical stimulation—to relieve pain. Physical therapists will teach you exercises to strengthen your back and improve flexibility. They will encourage you to stay as active as possible since staying in bed often makes back pain worse.

Studies have shown that physical therapy for low back pain can reduce the need for subsequent medical care and will provide substantial cost savings. In a study of 32,070 patients with low back pain, those who saw a physical therapist early in their treatment saved an average of $2,736 in medical costs. An analysis of more than 750,000 patients with low back pain in the US military reported that not only was physical therapy cost-effective, it also reduced the use of opioid medications, spinal injections, surgery, and other treatments.

Chiropractic and Osteopathic Manipulation

Spinal manipulation is the most popular alternative treatment for back pain. Seventy-four percent of people who used alternative therapies for low back pain reported seeing a chiropractor. Two-thirds of them said that they had received "great benefit" from the treatment. My own experience attests to this. When my daughter was eight months old, I developed severe back pain from carrying her around on my hip. One visit to the chiropractor, now one of my dearest friends, and I was saved.

Research has confirmed that spinal manipulation is effective for acute, subacute, and chronic low back pain, as well as for joint pains and headaches. A review of twenty-six trials of spinal manipulation in patients who had suffered from low back pain for twelve weeks or more reported that it was as effective as standard medical care or physical therapy.

Chiropractors attend four-year chiropractic medical schools and are licensed by individual states. They adjust and manipulate the spine to relieve pain and help the body to function better. Spinal manipulation is also carried out by other practitioners including osteopathic and naturopathic physicians, physical therapists, and some medical doctors.

Massage, Exercise, and Yoga

Massage is also very helpful in relieving back pain. Self-massage is one approach. My husband has low back pain on occasion, most recently after I persuaded him to take me out dancing and he overdid it. But he received a tip from an osteopathic doctor friend years ago that he still finds quite useful. He lies on his back with his knees up and feet on the floor. He then places a very tightly rolled strip from a washcloth secured with a rubber band—about an inch and a half in diameter and three inches long—under his spine. It feels awkward for a moment or two until he relaxes into it. After a few minutes in each location, he moves the cloth up or down to another spot on his spine and relaxes into it.

Professional massage of various types will relax back muscles and alleviate pain. The most common is Swedish massage, but most practitioners today use a variety of methods. A study of 401 patients with chronic back pain compared massage therapy with usual care—ice, heat, and OTC pain relievers. After ten weeks, those receiving massage therapy used less medication, missed less work, and had better scores on pain and physical functioning questionnaires.

Exercise reduces low back pain and improves the long-term functioning of people who suffer from it. Walking on a level surface for ten to twenty minutes at a time several times a day can help alleviate acute back pain, while lying down or sitting in the same position for more than thirty minutes can aggravate it. Exercise also is effective in preventing low back pain, according to a meta-analysis of twenty-three studies. Basic exercises for low back pain along with diagrams explaining them can be found at: uhs.berkeley.edu/sites/default/files/lowbackpain.pdf.

Yoga is a type of exercise that combines stretching, breathing techniques, and relaxation. In a study of people with chronic low back pain, those taking yoga classes over a twelve-week period had greater improvement in back function than those who received usual care. In a similar study, both yoga and stretching exercises led by a physical therapist resulted in less pain, better functioning, and reduced use of medication when compared to a self-care handbook recommending exercises and lifestyle changes to control pain.

Acupuncture and Homeopathy

Acupuncture is another treatment that should be considered for low back pain. In an analysis of twenty-nine trials involving nearly 18,000 patients, acupuncture was effective for several types of chronic pain, including low back, neck, knee, and headache. This was in comparison to patients receiving usual care as well as those receiving "sham acupuncture," an experimental design in which acupuncture needles are used but are not inserted into the correct places.

In Germany, studies have shown that acupuncture is cost-effective and better than standard care (physical therapy, exercise, and OTC pain medications) for back pain. The German government decided in 2006 to include reimbursement for acupuncture treatment of chronic low back pain in the social health-care system. In the United States, some insurance companies will pay for treatment with acupuncture, but others will not.

Homeopathy also shows promise in the treatment of low back pain. In another German study, 129 adults who had suffered from low back pain for an average of more than nine years were treated with individualized homeopathic medicines over the course of the next two years. At the end of that time, they experienced significant reductions in the severity of their symptoms, their quality of life improved, and their use of conventional health services and drugs decreased markedly.

Cognitive Behavioral Therapy and Mindfulness-based Stress Reduction

Chronic pain often has a psychological component due to the constant stress and discomfort. This can exacerbate the problem, leading to a downward spiral of pain, depression, more pain, and so forth. Because of this, psychological therapies such as cognitive behavioral therapy (CBT) and mindfulness meditation have been used to treat low back pain with some success.

In a meta-analysis of twenty-three studies of over 6,000 people with chronic low back pain, CBT yielded long-term improvements in pain, disability, and quality of life. CBT and mindfulness-based stress reduction, which combines meditation with yoga, were both better than usual care in a study that evaluated pain and functioning of people with chronic low back pain.

TENS Units

When we were trying to find an alternative to morphine for Arlyn's back pain, her physician suggested that she try using a TENS unit. TENS stands for transcutaneous electrical nerve stimulation, a method by which low-level electrical current is applied to relieve pain. The battery-operated unit is worn on a belt around the lower back and sends current directly to the skin. There are different theories about how this works and studies have failed to verify its effectiveness. Some say that the electrical current stimulates nerve fibers, which then block other pain signals. Others think it may activate endorphins, the body's innate pain relievers. TENS units are available online for under $50. Use of a TENS unit is relatively safe, but you should check with your doctor before trying one.

NECK PAIN

Neck pain has many of the same causes as back pain—muscle strains, ruptured or bulging vertebral disks, osteoarthritis, and osteoporosis. It can be caused by poor posture, sitting too long at the computer, or sleeping in a bad position. The neck is particularly vulnerable to injury from a sudden jolt, also known as whiplash. In a government survey, 15 percent of adults reported having had neck pain in the previous three months.

You can reduce your risk of neck pain by following several commonsense measures. Make sure you have a comfortable pillow and try to sleep mainly on your back. (I use a contoured memory-foam pillow that gives extra support to the neck area and feels oh-so-good when I first lie down at night.) Your computer screen should be directly at eye level and if you spend a lot of time on your phone, use earbuds or headphones to reduce neck strain. For good posture, do not allow your head to slant forward in front of your shoulders, which puts stress on the lower neck. If you carry a purse or a handbag, alternate which shoulder you strap it across, or better yet, use a backpack instead.

Managing Neck Pain without Drugs

When you feel your neck starting to feel tight, do some simple exercises. Slowly move your head forward, bringing your chin to your chest and then all the way back so that you are looking up at the ceiling. Then bring your head back to the center and slowly move it side to side, bringing each ear down toward your shoulders. Finally, starting with your chin at your chest, slowly roll your head all the way around in one direction, then reverse and go in the other direction. Do each of these exercises three times and you will feel your muscles relax.

Many of the same nondrug strategies used for back pain are also beneficial for neck pain. Physical therapy, chiropractic, acupuncture, massage, and yoga are common treatments, as well as TENS units applied to the neck. A British study evaluated acupuncture and the Alexander Technique—a process that helps to realign posture and relieve muscle tension in the body—in patients with chronic neck pain. Researchers reported significant decreases in pain and disability after one year using either one of these therapies compared to those on standard medication and physical therapy.

OSTEOARTHRITIS

Osteoarthritis (OA), or degenerative joint disease, affects over 30 million Americans. More than one-third of the population aged sixty or older has X-ray evidence of knee osteoarthritis, although only 12 percent report symptoms. Osteoarthritis is caused by the age-associated breakdown and loss of the soft tissue—cartilage—that provides a cushion between the bones in a joint. Without cartilage, bones grind against each other, causing pain and inflammation. Joint pain and stiffness of OA are often worse in the morning or after resting. Sometimes joints swell after too much activity. Bone spurs or nodules can occur, most typically on the finger joints or at the base of the big toe, forming a bunion.

The most common sites of OA are the hip, knee, and fingers, but it can also occur in the spine, as we have already seen. Obesity is the second most common risk factor for OA after aging, due to extra stress being put on the hips and knees. People who have been active in sports such as soccer, weight lifting, or skiing are more prone to developing OA of the knee, as are those who have worked in jobs requiring heavy labor, like construction or agriculture. There appears to be a genetic component to OA, as it seems to run in families. Injuries to joints can also lead to OA.

Managing Osteoarthritis without Drugs

The keys to preventing and treating osteoarthritis pain without medication are physical activity, weight management, and nutrition. Tai chi and certain supplements also can reduce the symptoms of OA in some people.

Physical Activity

Staying active is an important part of keeping your joints supple and pain-free. The best exercises are those that do not put a lot of stress on your joints, such as walking on level surfaces, using a stationary bike, and swimming. If you have knee or hip pain, avoid jogging and other intense aerobic activities that put extra pressure on these joints. It is also important to do exercises that strengthen the muscles around your joints, which will provide added support. Exercise will also help you to reduce any excess weight you might have.

There is good research backing up these recommendations. One review reported that aerobic, muscle strengthening, water exercises, and tai chi all helped to improve pain and joint function in people with OA. A meta-analysis of ninety-one different studies of people with knee OA reported that resistance training—using weights, bands, or exercise machines, as well as walking, cycling, swimming, tai chi, and yoga are all effective for reducing symptoms and improving knee function.

There are a lot of good exercise choices to consider and it is important to find one that you enjoy. You might have trouble sticking with an exercise program in the beginning, but you should persevere. Some people find it easier to stay in a program if it is a group session supervised by a physical therapist or other professional. Having an exercise partner is another way to stay motivated.

Weight Management

You may be tired of my emphasis on weight loss as a way to solve your health problems, but with osteoarthritis of the hip or knees, losing those extra pounds can have a major impact on how you feel. If you are overweight, there is more stress on your hip and knee joints, making it more likely that the cartilage will break down. Studies show that dropping just ten to fifteen pounds can alleviate pain, improve function, and may help to avoid a hip or knee replacement. Knee replacement surgery, I recently heard on the radio, is the new tonsillectomy for baby boomers, with at least one million procedures in 2015 alone.

Even losing only a few pounds will do you some good. In a fascinating study that looked at weight loss and mechanical stress on the knee, researchers reported that for every pound lost, four pounds less pressure was exerted on the knee joint with each step. They calculated that for someone losing ten pounds, each knee would be subjected to 48,000 pounds less load per mile walked.

Another study found a direct relationship between weight gain or loss and knee pain, as well as the actual amount of cartilage lost in the knees.

Losing that ten to fifteen pounds isn't easy, but it can be done. Diet and exercise together is the best plan. In a study of 454 overweight or obese sedentary people aged fifty-five or older with knee OA, a steady program of diet and exercise over eighteen months resulted in more than a twenty-pound average weight loss as well as a significant decrease in knee pain. Calories were restricted to 1,200 per day and participants exercised for one hour three times a week. The exercise program consisted of fifteen minutes of aerobic walking, twenty minutes of strength training, another fifteen minutes of walking, and then a ten-minute cool down. Those using diet alone did not have as much improvement.

Nutrition

Since much of the pain of osteoarthritis is due to inflammation, eating foods that reduce the inflammatory process can be helpful in managing this disease. Multiple studies have shown that diets high in fiber, healthy oils (omega-3 fatty acids), and fruits and vegetables and low in sugars, starchy carbohydrates, and unhealthy oils (omega-6 fatty acids) can reduce inflammation.

Turmeric, a yellow-colored spice, has been used in traditional Chinese and Indian medicine to treat arthritis for centuries. The active ingredient—curcumin—is an anti-inflammatory similar to COX-2 inhibitors such as *Celebrex*. In a study of 107 patients with knee osteoarthritis, those receiving 2 grams per day of curcumin extract for six weeks had the same amount of improvement in pain and knee function as those taking 800 milligrams of ibuprofen daily. Ginger acts in the same way and studies have shown that ginger extract can significantly reduce knee pain when compared to a placebo.

Omega-3 oils, such as flaxseed and fish oils, have been shown to reduce joint pain in people with rheumatoid arthritis, a chronic inflammatory disease affecting many joints, especially the fingers and toes. In a meta-analysis of seventeen different studies, supplementation with omega-3s for three to four months reduced joint pain, morning stiffness, number of painful joints, and use of nonsteroidal anti-inflammatory drugs. The dosages used in these studies were 3,000 to 4,000 mg of combined omega-3 oils, which can usually be found in 6,000 to 8,000 mg of fish oil. There is preliminary evidence that omega-3s also can be beneficial for inflammatory pain associated with osteoarthritis, but more research needs to be done.

Tai Chi

Tai chi is another option for osteoarthritis that you might want to explore. It is a practice that combines slow, gentle movements with meditation and deep breathing. It is usually done in a group setting two to three times a week. Tai chi has gained popularity as a treatment for knee osteoarthritis since several studies have reported that it can relieve pain and increase physical functioning without the side effects of common over-the-counter pain relievers. A 2016 meta-analysis found that for people with OA, practicing tai chi for at least six weeks resulted in significant improvements in pain. Those who practiced for longer had even better results.

Another 2016 study compared 204 patients aged forty or older with knee OA who were randomized to either practice tai chi practice or receive physical therapy. After twelve weeks, both groups had less pain and stiffness and the improvements lasted for one year. There were no significant differences between the two groups in physical functioning and use of medication, but the tai chi group showed greater improvements in quality-of-life scores and had less depression.

Glucosamine and Chondroitin

Many people with osteoarthritis are helped by supplements containing glucosamine and chondroitin, which can be purchased OTC in the United States. Both of these substances are found naturally in joint cartilage, although supplements containing them are manufactured from animal cartilage or synthesized in a laboratory. Because they are not regulated as drugs, the dosages and quality of the supplements vary among different products.

Recent research suggests that the combination of glucosamine and chondroitin is effective in reducing knee pain, especially in people with moderate-to-severe pain. A 2006 study funded by the National Institutes of Health found significant relief of knee pain in patients with moderate-to-severe pain when the combination was compared to a placebo.

Two newer studies have bolstered these results. In an Australian study, researchers reported a significant reduction in joint space narrowing in those taking glucosamine and chondroitin, suggesting that they might slow the degenerative process of OA. Researchers calculated that if fourteen people took these supplements for two years, one knee replacement surgery could be prevented within the next five years.

The second study was done in Europe, where the combination of these two supplements is a prescription medicine. A product containing glucosamine (500 milligrams) and chondroitin (400 milligrams) taken three times a day was as effective as the anti-inflammatory celecoxib (*Celebrex*) in people with moderate-to-severe knee pain. After six months, there were no differences between the two groups—both had a 50 percent decrease in pain as well as improvements in stiffness and overall knee function.

If you decide to take a glucosamine-chondroitin supplement, you might try dosages similar to those used in the European study. Not only does this combination have the potential to give you sufficient pain relief, it also can slow down the aging process of your joints. Combining it with other nondrug approaches or OTC pain medications might give you the best result. These supplements appear to be safe, although not much is known about their long-term side effects. Some people experience mild gastrointestinal symptoms, which can be prevented by taking them with food. Don't take chondroitin sulfate with aspirin, as it can contribute to bleeding problems.

NONDRUG MANAGEMENT OF CHRONIC PAIN

- Physical therapy
- Weight management
- Physical activity
- Chiropractic and osteopathic manipulation
- TENS unit
- Massage, tai chi, Alexander Technique, and yoga
- Acupuncture and homeopathy
- Cognitive behavioral therapy and mindfulness stress reduction
- Anti-inflammatory diet, curcumin, ginger, omega-3 oils
- Glucosamine and chondroitin

MEDICATIONS FOR BACK, NECK, AND OSTEOARTHRITIS PAIN

There is a hierarchy of medicines to consider in treating back, neck, or OA pain, ranging from simple over-the-counter (OTC) pain relievers to prescription COX-2 inhibitors, steroid injections, and opioids.

Over-the-Counter Pain Relievers and Anti-inflammatories

Sometimes nondrug treatments are not enough to give sufficient pain relief, in which case you should first consider OTC medications. There are two main classes of these—simple pain relievers and nonsteroidal anti-inflammatory drugs (NSAIDs). These can be as effective as prescription pain medications, although they have significant side effects when used in high doses or over the long term. Topical creams and rubs such as capsaicin (*Capzasin*), trolamine salicylate (*Aspercreme*), methyl salicylate (*Bengay*), and menthol preparations can be useful in providing temporary pain relief.

Acetaminophen (Tylenol)

Acetaminophen (*Tylenol*) is the most common pain reliever recommended for back and joint pain. Known as paracetamol in Europe, it does not have the gastrointestinal side effects that accompany NSAIDs. It is extremely inexpensive, costing only pennies per dose. Also used to treat fever, acetaminophen is often combined with other over-the-counter medications for headaches, colds, and even sleep problems. It is also combined into a single pill with prescription pain relievers, such as oxycodone (*Percocet*). Acetaminophen with codeine is the number one prescribed generic drug in the United States.

While it is considered a mainstay of treatment for back pain and osteoarthritis, I was surprised to find two recent studies that cast doubt on the effectiveness of acetaminophen for these ailments. In an analysis of thirteen studies comparing acetaminophen with placebo, researchers concluded that even in doses of up to 4,000 milligrams per day, it was ineffective for the treatment of low back pain and provided only minimal short-term benefit for people with osteoarthritis. A similar analysis on low back pain also reported that acetaminophen was no better than placebo for pain relief, nor did it appear to provide any improvements in quality of life, physical functioning, and sleep.

We need to keep in mind that these results do not mean that acetaminophen is ineffective for everyone, just on average when considering pain relief in these study populations. Also, placebo has been shown to cause natural pain relieving opioids to be produced in the body, so an effect equivalent to placebo does not mean no effect.

Acetaminophen is relatively safe when taken in low doses—no more than 2,000 milligrams per day for women and 3,000 for men. The most serious side effect is liver failure. A daily dose of 4,000 milligrams per day—the maximum amount recommended on the label—has been associated with liver damage when taken for only fourteen days in healthy people. Acetaminophen causes almost half of all acute liver failure cases in the United States and acetaminophen overdose is the leading reason for calls to poison control centers—more than 100,000 each year. It also accounts for more than 33,000 hospitalizations, and an estimated 300 deaths each year. People taking several different combination medications containing acetaminophen may be unaware of the total amount they are taking, making them more at risk.

Other side effects of acetaminophen are more troubling than experts previously thought, especially when taken in higher doses. A review of the long-term effects of acetaminophen reported evidence of increased mortality (death rates), more heart attacks, strokes, coronary heart disease, ulcers, gastrointestinal (GI) bleeding, and kidney damage in people taking them. Researchers also reported strong evidence of a dose-response relationship, in which those taking higher doses had increased risks of these adverse events.

Nonsteroidal Anti-inflammatory Drugs (NSAIDs)

You have no doubt taken one or more of these common drugs during your lifetime, if not within the past few weeks. Aspirin, ibuprofen (*Advil, Motrin*), and naproxen (*Naprosyn, Aleve*) are the most common over-the-counter NSAIDs. More than 30 million people use NSAIDs every day, and they account for 60 percent of the US over-the-counter pain-relief market. In addition to relieving pain, they also have anti-inflammatory properties, which makes them especially useful for people with chronic pain.

An analysis of seventeen different placebo-controlled studies of people with chronic knee pain showed that NSAIDs offered similar pain relief as opioid pain medications, without the risk of addiction. Let me say that again—*NSAIDs offered similar pain relief as opioid pain medications*. NSAIDs work by blocking the enzymes COX-1 and COX-2, important in the production of prostaglandins, which promote inflammation. Prostaglandins are also important in blood clotting mechanisms and some of them protect the stomach lining from excess acid.

Common side effects of NSAIDs include nausea, vomiting, diarrhea, constipation, rash, dizziness, and headache. The most serious adverse effects are peptic ulcers and GI bleeding, which result in more than 100,000 hospital admissions annually in the United States and as many as 16,500 deaths. Risk factors for GI bleeding from NSAIDs include:

- age sixty-five and older

- history of peptic ulcer disease
- taking more than one NSAID at the same time, including low-dose aspirin
- taking any one of the following other medications with an NSAID: anticoagulants, corticosteroids, SSRI antidepressants, anti-platelet drugs
- alcoholic drinks

While aspirin is used to prevent heart disease, non-aspirin NSAIDs have been associated with a two- to threefold increased risk of heart attacks and strokes, most likely due to their effect on blood clotting. The FDA issued a safety announcement in July 2015 advising patients taking non-aspirin NSAIDs to immediately seek medical care if they have symptoms of heart attack or stroke. The risk of heart attack is highest in the first month of taking NSAIDs and with higher doses.

Long-term use of high doses of NSAIDs can damage the kidneys, leading to high blood pressure and kidney failure. People who already have kidney problems are more at risk for this as well as those who take more than one type of OTC pain medication or who take more than six doses a day of NSAIDs for three years or more. NSAIDs can also cause severe allergic reactions, especially in people with asthma, who should avoid taking them. Disturbing new evidence suggests that combining NSAIDs with antidepressants increases the risk of bleeding inside the brain.

Because of the risks of long-term side effects, the FDA recommends taking the lowest effective dose possible of NSAIDs for the shortest amount of time. Maximum recommended daily doses of over-the-counter NSAIDs for adults are: aspirin, 4,000 milligrams; ibuprofen, 1,200 milligrams; and naproxen, 660 milligrams. Lower doses are safer, however, especially for smaller people.

Prescription Pain Medications

There are several types of prescription pain medications—topical NSAIDs, COX-2 inhibitors, corticosteroids, and opioids.

Topical NSAIDs

Topical diclofenac (*Voltaren, Flector*) is an NSAID that is applied directly to the skin of the painful area in the form of a gel, patch, or liquid solution. It is available only by prescription and costs $200 to $400 for a month's supply, depending on the preparation and how frequently you use it. Topical NSAIDs should reduce the risk of GI bleeding, heart attacks, and strokes, since there is less of the drug circulating in the bloodstream. While this makes sense, it has not been definitely proven. Studies have shown that these topical agents are as effective as oral NSAIDs when compared to a placebo. Their main side effect is skin irritation at the site to which they are applied.

COX-2 Inhibitors

COX-2 inhibitors are a relatively new class of NSAIDs that do not have the gastrointestinal side effects of other NSAIDs. This is because they inhibit only the COX-2 enzyme, which does not block the prostaglandins that protect the stomach lining.

Celecoxib (*Celebrex*) is the only COX-2 inhibitor now available in the United States and only by prescription. It is no more effective in reducing pain than the over-the-counter NSAIDs, but is much more expensive—costing an average of $200 to $300 for a month's supply compared to $4 to $10 for generic ibuprofen, aspirin, or naproxen. It may be the best choice if you have a history of ulcers or gastrointestinal bleeding, although acetaminophen is less costly and also carries less risk of these side effects.

The main problem with the COX-2 inhibitors is that they throw off the balance between the two COX enzymes, making blood clotting—leading to heart attacks and strokes—much more likely. Two early COX-2 inhibitors, *Vioxx* and *Bextra*, are no longer sold due to this. You might recall that *Vioxx* caused upward of 100,000 heart attacks before it was taken off the market. COX-2 inhibitors carry a higher risk of heart attacks and strokes than over-the-counter NSAIDs, although high-dose ibuprofen also has been reported to be associated with these problems.

Corticosteroids

Corticosteroids are anti-inflammatory drugs that can provide relief of pain for inflamed joints. Oral corticosteroids are not usually given for chronic pain, but doctors sometimes inject cortisone into the spine or joints for temporary relief of persistent pain. Unfortunately, these injections can cause thinning of joint cartilage as well as accelerate its breakdown since they allow people to avoid the pain that would normally keep them from putting further strain on the joints. A study comparing steroid with saline (a sterile salt solution) injections in the knee joints of patients with osteoarthritis found no difference in knee pain but more cartilage loss after two years in those receiving the steroid injections.

Opioid Pain Relievers

Opium, derived from the seed-pod of poppies, has been used for thousands of years for the treatment of pain and psychological distress. Until aspirin was synthesized at the end of the nineteenth century, opium was the only medicine available to relieve pain. Painkillers produced from opium—also called narcotics—include morphine, hydromorphone (*Dilaudid*), codeine, hydrocodone (*Vicodin*), oxycodone (*OxyContin*), and fentanyl (*Duragesic*).

Opioids reduce the number of pain signals sent to the brain and switch off the brain's reaction to them. This dulls your perception of pain and also calms your response to it. For more than thirty years, opioids have been used to treat chronic pain, yet there is little proof of their safety and effectiveness for long-term treatment. This is disturbing, considering that the potential for abuse of these highly addictive drugs is great and thousands of people fall victim to this abuse every year.

Despite their reputation for being strong painkillers, several studies show that opioids are no better than NSAIDs in relieving pain. A meta-analysis of the effectiveness of opioids for chronic noncancer pain found little difference in pain relief between them and other drugs. Improvements in physical function were actually better in those receiving the nonopioid drugs. A different meta-analysis, this one of opioids for chronic low back pain, reported that they provided better pain relief than a placebo but were no better than NSAIDs. And a meta-analysis of opioids for knee and hip pain reported that they were minimally better than placebo but that ten patients would need to be treated for only one to benefit.

The perception that opioids are more effective than other painkillers could be due to their greater ability to relieve the emotional distress of pain. It is this benefit that most likely leads people to become more and more dependent and finally addicted to these drugs. In my own experience of taking a narcotic pain reliever after surgery many years ago, I remember being aware of having pain but not feeling disturbed by it.

The major physical side effects of opioids are constipation, sleepiness, and nausea. Constipation can be severe, as we saw in my mother-in-law Arlyn's case, and does not improve over time. High doses of opioids can cause depression of the respiratory system and should not be given to people with chronic lung disease. Opioids can also increase the risk of depression when taken for more than thirty days. The FDA recently issued a safety announcement warning that taking opioids with antidepressants increases the risk of serotonin syndrome, as well as problems with the adrenal gland and sex hormones.

The most dangerous adverse effects of opioid pain medications are unintentional overdoses, many in people who started out with a valid prescription for chronic pain. Research shows that more than four million people use painkillers for nonmedical reasons and that four out of five new heroin users started out by misusing prescription painkillers. Heroin is now less expensive than illicit prescription opioids. Fentanyl, which is even stronger than heroin, is now being mixed with heroin and sold on the street. In my hometown of Huntington, West Virginia, there were twenty-six overdoses in a four-hour period in August 2016. Fortunately, thanks to the efforts of emergency responders, nobody died.

Alarmed over the epidemic of opioid drug overdoses, the CDC has issued new guidelines to doctors for opioid prescribing. "For the vast majority of patients, the known, serious, and all too often fatal risks [of opioids] far outweigh the unproven and transient benefits, and there are safer alternatives," said Dr. Tom Frieden, the former director of the CDC. The new guidelines state that opioids should *not* be the first-line therapy for chronic pain, and that clinicians should first consider nonopioid pain relievers or nonpharmacological options such as exercise and cognitive behavioral therapy.

Type of Pain Medicine	Examples (Brand Name)	How They Work	Possible Side Effects
OTC analgesics	Acetaminophen (*Tylenol*); Paracetamol (*Panadol, Calpol*)	Weak inhibitor of prostaglandins with some similarities to COX-2 inhibitors	Nausea, vomiting, and constipation; liver damage and acute liver failure in high doses
Nonsteroidal anti-inflammatories (NSAIDs)	Aspirin (*Ecotrin, Bayer*); Ibuprofen (*Advil, Motrin, Nuprin*); Naproxen (*Aleve, Naprosyn, Anaprox*)	Decrease inflammation, pain, and fever by inhibiting COX-1 and COX-2 enzymes needed to make prostaglandins	Nausea, vomiting, diarrhea or constipation, rash, dizziness, and headache; gastrointestinal ulcers and bleeding; increased risk of heart attacks and strokes
Topical NSAIDs	Diclofenac (*Voltaren, Flector*)	Decrease inflammation, pain, and fever by inhibiting COX-1 and COX-2 enzymes needed to make prostaglandins	Local skin irritation; less risk of systemic adverse effects

COX-2 inhibitors	Celecoxib (*Celebrex*)	Inhibit prostaglandins made from COX-2 enzymes only	Same as NSAIDs except no gastrointestinal risk but more risk of heart attacks and strokes
Opioids	Morphine, Codeine; Hydromorphone (*Dilaudid*); Hydrocodone (*Vicodin*); Oxycodone (*OxyContin*, *Percocet*); Fentanyl (*Duragesic*, *Actiq*, *Abstral*)	Reduce the number of pain signals sent to the brain and decrease the brain's response to pain	Constipation, nausea, sleepiness, and depression; serotonin syndrome with other drugs; addiction, death by overdose

DO YOU REALLY NEED THAT PAIN PILL?

Dealing with chronic pain is not easy. But as you have seen, there are several nondrug approaches that not only can help manage your pain, but also will keep you healthier in the long run. Staying active is the most important. Walking, swimming, or doing yoga, tai chi, or other gentle exercises can help you stay flexible and improve your pain and level of functioning. Keeping your weight down will take some of the load off your back, hip, and knee joints and help to relieve pain.

Physical therapy, massage, and spinal manipulation have all been shown to alleviate pain, along with alternative therapies such as acupuncture and homeopathy. TENS units and supplements such as glucosamine and chondroitin also have a place in pain management as do ways to cope with the emotional components of pain, like behavioral therapy and meditation.

If one or more of these is not enough to eliminate your pain or keep it at a minimal level, the next step is to take an OTC pain medication. Which one you take depends on your overall health and risk factors. Acetaminophen is the safest medicine, as long as you don't have liver problems. Using that along with a topical NSAID such as diclofenac is recommended as the first line of treatment for chronic pain by National Institute for Health and Care Excellence in the United Kingdom. Another OTC option is the combination of acetaminophen and aspirin, found in *Excedrin*, which also contains caffeine and is more often taken for headaches.

Oral NSAIDs should be the next step if acetaminophen and topical NSAIDs don't provide sufficient relief. OTC aspirin, ibuprofen, and naproxen are inexpensive and have been shown to provide pain relief similar to opioids. You should consider taking a COX-2 inhibitor only if you have a history of ulcers or GI bleeding, since this class of drugs causes an increased risk of heart attacks and strokes.

Opioids have no place in routine therapy for chronic noncancer pain, according to the new CDC guidelines, since they are no better than other pain relievers and carry the risk of abuse, addiction, overdose, and death. When opioids are prescribed for acute pain from an injury or after surgery, the CDC recommends that prescriptions be limited to a three- to seven-day supply. Hopefully these new guidelines will help reduce the overprescribing of these dangerous drugs, as doctors become more knowledgeable about other options for treating pain.

If you or a family member suffers from chronic pain, I hope that you will use the information in this chapter to find a safe and effective solution for your problem. There are many alternatives that can help you to avoid taking that pain pill.

Chapter 8

High Blood Pressure

High blood pressure (hypertension) is the main risk factor for heart attacks and strokes, two of the three leading causes of death in the United States. According to the CDC, about 75 million adults in the United States have hypertension—nearly one in three. The yearly cost of this disorder—for health-care services, medications, and missed days of work—is estimated to be $46 billion, more than 1 percent of the nation's total health-care budget. Nearly half of this, $20.4 billion, is spent on drugs alone. Clearly this is an important and costly public health problem. But do all of these people really have hypertension? And do all of them need to take drugs?

DO YOU REALLY HAVE HIGH BLOOD PRESSURE?

Blood pressure is the force of blood pushing against your artery walls. If it is too high, it can damage your arteries, sometimes leading to heart attacks and strokes. In determining whether or not you have hypertension, two blood pressure measurements are taken—the systolic, the peak pressure when your heart contracts, and the diastolic, when the heart relaxes. An inflatable arm cuff using a scale called "millimeters of mercury" (mm Hg) is used to measure these pressures. The upper number is your systolic pressure and the bottom number is the diastolic. A blood pressure reading of 120/80 or below is considered normal, above 120/80 to 140/90 is borderline (also called *prehypertension*), and more than 140/90 is classified as hypertension.

Many people are diagnosed with hypertension who don't really have it and are placed on medication that they don't really need. This happens for several reasons. Often the diagnosis of high blood pressure is based on only one reading, taken in the doctor's office. Blood pressure is dynamic and changes throughout the day. One reading is only a snapshot of a more complicated overall picture. Expert guidelines recommend that blood pressure be taken after sitting quietly for five to ten minutes with the feet placed firmly on the ground.

It is well known that many people experience what is called "white coat syndrome," whereby the stress of being in a doctor's office is enough to push their blood pressure up. Couple this with rushing to get there and then becoming upset at spending too much time waiting and it is understandable that a blood pressure measurement might be too high. A caffeinated drink or smoking within the previous half hour can also falsely elevate blood pressure.

It has been estimated by the Agency for Healthcare Research and Quality that 15 to 30 percent of people diagnosed with hypertension in the doctor's office have normal blood pressure. The US Preventive Services Task Force (USPSTF) recommends obtaining measurements outside of the office setting to confirm the diagnosis before starting medication. This can be done using an ambulatory monitor that checks blood pressure periodically and is worn for twenty-four hours, considered the "gold standard" for blood pressure measurement. However, it is bulky to wear and expensive—about $200 for the test, although paid for by most insurance. More convenient is home blood pressure monitoring using an inexpensive electronic device available at most drugstores. Checking your blood pressure twice daily for about a week, at approximately the same times in the morning and evening will give you a better idea of whether or not you have high blood pressure.

This is what happened to Dawn, who was running late the day of her doctor's appointment for an annual exam. She had just gotten off the phone with a high-maintenance client when her three-year-old dumped a bowl of cereal on the floor. After cleaning up the mess and dropping off her daughter at preschool, Dawn stopped at a drive-through for a cup of espresso. When she got to the clinic, the parking lot was full so she had to park on the street half a block away and rush to the building.

By the time Dawn arrived in the waiting room, her name was called. The medical assistant weighed her in and then took her into an exam room to check her blood pressure. "Oh my," she told Dawn, "your blood pressure is 160 over 95—way too high!" Dawn waited quietly in the exam room for ten minutes and calmed down before her doctor came in and checked her blood pressure again. This time the reading was perfect—120/80.

WHO SHOULD TAKE MEDICINE FOR HIGH BLOOD PRESSURE?

There is no consensus about when people should start taking medication for high blood pressure. As with other conditions, expert panels are convened to make recommendations for doctors to follow. And as with other panels, many of these experts are in the employ of the companies that manufacture these medications. One of the members of the most recent group issuing guidelines for hypertension treatment reported potential conflicts of interest from seventeen different pharmaceutical and device manufacturers, including membership on the advisory boards of five companies and consulting fees from ten of them.

Sixty percent of people with high blood pressure have what is considered *mild hypertension*, with blood pressures in the 140/90 to 160/100 range. According to the guidelines of several expert groups, these people should take medication, although some recommend a systolic of 150 to start therapy in people over age sixty. However, the co-chair of a group issuing guidelines for hypertension treatment said in an interview that "physicians can typically give low-to-moderate-risk individuals a few months with lifestyle changes to determine whether they're having an impact on blood pressure."

There is little evidence that people with mild hypertension who take medication have improved health. A review of several studies of otherwise healthy people with mild hypertension found no difference in the number of deaths, heart attacks, or strokes in those taking medications compared to those taking a placebo. Nearly 10 percent of the patients who were taking medications dropped out of the studies because of adverse side effects.

In a 2014 editorial in the highly regarded *British Medical Journal*, two hypertension specialists wrote that millions of people around the world are being treated unnecessarily with drugs for mild hypertension, exposing them to more potential harm than good and wasting health-care resources. They went on to say that "for patients with mild hypertension, the focus on drug treatment reduces emphasis on lifestyle changes. Unlike drug treatment, lifestyle changes are free of side effects and provide benefits beyond reduced blood pressure." As we will see later, there are significant side effects with many of the most popular medications for hypertension, especially for those aged sixty-five or older.

MANAGING HIGH BLOOD PRESSURE WITHOUT DRUGS

Many doctors are quicker to write a prescription for high blood pressure medication than to advise their patients to make healthy lifestyle changes. This could be due to the changes in the 2014 hypertension guidelines. The previous guidelines, published in 2004, recommended that *lifestyle modifications* should be the initial treatment strategy for lowering blood pressure. The newer ones recommend that *pharmacological treatment* be initiated at blood pressures of 150/90 in those over age sixty and at 140/90 in younger adults. The 2014 guidelines go into great detail about the various medications that can be used to keep blood pressure below these thresholds but include only a brief mention about lifestyle changes toward the end of the document.

This change in emphasis is unfortunate, since there is ample evidence that eating a healthy diet, exercising, and cutting down on salt can lower blood pressure enough for many people with mild hypertension to avoid taking medication. An expert panel made up mostly of nutritionists, exercise physiologists, and epidemiologists reviewed dozens of studies about lifestyle management of heart disease published between 1998 and 2011 and found that:

- A diet consisting of vegetables, fruits, low-fat dairy products, whole grains, poultry, fish, and nuts that is low in sweets, sugar-sweetened beverages, and red meats was found to lower blood pressure by **5–6 mm Hg systolic and 3 mm Hg diastolic**.

- Decreasing salt intake to about 1 teaspoon daily reduces BP by **3–4 mm Hg systolic and 1–2 mm Hg diastolic.**
- Moderate to vigorous aerobic activity lasting about forty minutes three to four times a week decreases systolic and diastolic BP on average by **2–5 mm Hg and 1–4 mm Hg**, respectively.

If you add all of these up, you could hypothetically lower your blood pressure by as much as **15 mm Hg systolic and 9 mm Hg diastolic** by making these lifestyle changes.

Heart-healthy diets

Diets that are effective in lowering blood pressure include the Mediterranean diet and the Dietary Approaches to Stop Hypertension (DASH) diet. DASH reduces blood pressure, sometimes in only a few weeks. The plan focuses on eating plenty of fruits, vegetables, and whole grains while lowering salt to no more than one teaspoon daily. It also includes low-fat dairy products, fish, poultry, beans, nuts, and vegetable oils. The DASH diet also encourages people to limit fatty meats, full-fat dairy products, oils such as coconut, palm kernel, and palm, sugar-sweetened beverages, and sweets.

The ability of the DASH diet to lower blood pressure was impressively demonstrated in a study of healthy but overweight people with borderline or mild hypertension—130 to 159 (systolic) / 85 to 99 (diastolic). These people were randomly assigned to one of three different treatment groups: the usual American diet, the DASH diet alone, or the DASH diet with exercise and weight reduction. After four months, the DASH diet alone brought down blood pressures by an average of 11.2 systolic and 7.5 diastolic.

This by itself could take many people out of the category needing treatment.

Even more beneficial were the results in the group that combined the DASH diet with exercise and weight reduction—decreases of on average 16 systolic and 10 diastolic. This is comparable, according to the authors, to what could be expected from taking a high dose antihypertension drug. In fact, they go even further, stating that "Similar BP reductions . . . have resulted in a lowering of stroke risk by approximately 40 percent and a reduction in ischemic heart disease events by about 25 percent."

Decreasing Salt (Sodium) Intake

The American Heart Association recommends no more than 2,300 mg—1 teaspoon—of table salt daily for most adults, with a lower goal of 1,500 mg for African Americans, those with heart disease, and those over age fifty. It might sound easy to cut down your intake of salt to one teaspoon a day, but it sneaks into your diet in many ways. More than 75 percent of the salt we consume—an average of 3,400 mg a day for Americans—comes from processed foods, those that have been changed from their original raw form. Processing a food often involves the use of added ingredients, including sodium-containing additives, to modify the flavor and act as a preservative.

If you walk into your kitchen and look at the nutritional labels on some of your food, you will see what I mean. Chips, salted nuts, and crackers are obvious sources of salt but bread, canned soup, canned vegetables, lunch meats, frozen and boxed meals, pizza, cereal, and salad dressing all have significant amounts of sodium. In a survey of common processed foods, bacon, hot dogs, pork sausage, Caesar salad dressing, sliced turkey breast, and barbecue sauce were found to have the highest sodium levels—more than 600 mg per serving.

Fast food and other restaurants are also sources of excess salt. A Quarter Pounder with Cheese at McDonald's has 1,190 mg of sodium and a medium order of french fries adds another 270 mg. Both of these together almost meet the total recommended daily amount of salt for people over age fifty. A study of twenty-six chain sit-down restaurants found that more than 80 percent of meals (breakfast, lunch, or dinner) contained more than 1,500 mg of sodium, while 50 percent of them had more than 2,300 mg.

The best way to avoid excess salt in your diet is to eat fresh, unprocessed foods, preferably home-cooked. Gradually decrease the amount of salt from your recipes, substituting herbs and spices, and remove the salt shaker from the table. Your food might taste bland at first, but after a few weeks your taste buds will adjust and you won't miss the salt. When shopping, try to avoid processed foods that list more than 200 mg sodium per serving on their nutritional labels. And at restaurants, go for food that is cooked to order and ask for salad dressings and sauces on the side.

Exercise

Exercise strengthens the heart, allowing it to pump more blood with less effort. This in turn lessens the force on your arteries, lowering your blood pressure. As we've already learned, regular aerobic exercise can reduce both the systolic and diastolic blood pressures by as much as 4 to 5 mm Hg. While this alone might not be enough to let you sidestep medication, in combination with other healthy lifestyle choices it might be the difference between taking a pill or not.

Any kind of moderate exercise—such as walking, biking, danc-ing, and swimming—done for thirty minutes four to five times weekly can be enough to improve your blood pressure. The intensity of exercise is considered moderate if it is enough for your heart rate and breathing to increase but you are still able to carry on a conversation. Taking the stairs instead of elevators, parking your car farther away from your destination, and taking a break every hour or so from sitting at a desk are other ways to increase your activity level.

In addition to aerobic exercise, practices such as yoga and tai chi can lower blood pressure. In a meta-analysis of twenty-eight studies of tai chi, participants were able to lower their blood pressures by an average of 6 mm Hg systolic and 3 mm Hg diastolic, which is comparable to first-line antihypertensive medicines. Those who practiced tai chi more than three times a week had a higher drop in systolic pressure, averaging 9.3 mm Hg.

Acupuncture

A preliminary study reported that electroacupuncture, a technique that uses low-intensity electric pulses through needles inserted in acupuncture points on the body, was effective in reducing blood pressure in 70 percent of patients treated over an eight-week period. Blood pressure was reduced by an average of 8 mm Hg systolic and 4 mm Hg diastolic. Other studies have demonstrated that acupuncture is effective in lowering blood pressure in patients who are already taking antihypertensive medication.

My husband, a retired family practice doctor, visited his internist for a routine checkup after he became eligible for Medicare. After sitting in a drafty room in a paper gown for fifteen minutes, he was already feeling stressed when a medical assistant came in, asked a battery of questions, and took his blood pressure. The next thing he knew, his doctor breezed in with the pronouncement, "Your blood pressure is 150/90—you have hypertension. Here is a prescription for a calcium channel blocker."

Dean had never been diagnosed with hypertension and knew enough that he held off on filling the prescription. He started monitoring his blood pressure at home and found that if he sat and relaxed for a few minutes before checking it, his blood pressure was borderline, around 140/85. He decided to cut back on salt and lost five pounds. He also began walking three times a week for thirty minutes. When he returned to his doctor for a follow-up appointment a month later, he purposely relaxed before his blood pressure was taken and it was 115/70, within the normal range. "Hypertension resolved!" said the internist, who was then surprised to find out that Dean hadn't taken the medication.

Other Ways to Control High Blood Pressure without Drugs

There are several other things you can do to reduce your blood pressure:

- Lose weight. A weight loss of only ten pounds can help decrease the load on your heart and reduce your blood pressure.
- Limit the amount of alcohol you drink. While small amounts of alcohol—one beer, a glass of wine, or a mixed drink for women, two of these for men—have been shown to reduce blood pressure, larger amounts can increase it.
- Limit your intake of caffeine. Caffeine has been shown to raise blood pressure shortly after drinking it, although its long-term effects on hypertension are unknown.
- Stop smoking. The nicotine in cigarettes will increase your blood pressure temporarily. Long-term damage to the walls of your arteries will cause them to

narrow, requiring more pressure to push the same amount of blood through them.

- Manage stress. It is well known that an acute episode of stress can cause a temporary spike in blood pressure due to the release of adrenaline, which causes arteries to constrict. Studies also have found that chronic stress is a likely cause of ongoing hypertension.

MEDICATIONS FOR HIGH BLOOD PRESSURE

If your blood pressure is higher than 140 to 150/90 and you are not able to lower it using lifestyle methods alone, taking a medication is your next option. Most experts agree that it is acceptable to start with any one of five different classes of drugs—a thiazide-type diuretic, beta-blocker, angiotensin-converting enzyme inhibitor (ACE), angiotensin receptor blocker (ARB), or calcium channel blocker (CCB), alone or in combination with each other. For the African American population, only thiazide diuretics and CCBs are recommended, since they seem to work better for unexplained reasons.

Thiazide Diuretics

The 2004 hypertension guidelines recommended starting with a thiazide diuretic, which was what I was taught in medical school. Common thiazide diuretics include hydrochlorothiazide (*Microzide*) and chlorthalidone (*Thalitone*). These drugs are available as generics, are inexpensive, and have a long track record of success, with side effects that are well known and manageable. They act by causing the kidneys to eliminate more sodium and water, which decreases blood volume and lowers the pressure inside the arteries. It is like turning down the faucet for a garden hose—less water going through the hose exerts less pressure on the inside of the hose. Hydrochlorothiazide remains one of the most popular medications for high blood pressure—it was the tenth most frequently prescribed generic drug in 2014, with nearly 50 million prescriptions.

As you might expect, diuretics increase the frequency of urination—more trips to the bathroom—which can be a bother. Also problematic is that some men on diuretics have difficulty with erections, due to lower blood volume. The biggest problem with these medicines is that they cause the body to lose potassium, which can lead to weakness, fatigue, and leg cramps. Most people on diuretics also take a potassium supplement to counteract this problem.

There are also diuretics that are called "potassium sparing"—they don't cause the body to excrete potassium. These medications, which include triamterene and amiloride, are not as effective in lowering blood pressure as other diuretics. They are usually used in combination with other agents.

Beta-Blockers

Beta-blockers are well known, inexpensive medications that have been, along with thiazide diuretics, the mainstay of hypertension treatment for several decades. Common beta-blockers are atenolol (*Tenormin*), metoprolol (*Lopressor*), and propranolol (*Inderal*). They work by blocking the action of the hormones norepinephrine and epinephrine (adrenaline) on the nervous system, causing the heart to beat less forcefully and opening up the blood vessels. They are especially useful for people with heart problems that also can be helped by these medicines—such as arrhythmias, chest pain (angina), and heart failure.

Beta-blockers also block the action of nerve receptors in other parts of the body, causing several side effects. These include depression, insomnia, erection problems, constipation, diarrhea, nausea and vomiting, dizziness, fatigue, and cold hands and feet. People with asthma or chronic lung disease should not take beta-blockers because they can cause air passages to constrict, triggering a severe asthma attack. It is important to taper off these drugs slowly if you need to discontinue them; stopping abruptly can increase the risk of a heart attack.

Angiotensin Converting Enzyme (ACE) Inhibitors

These medications block the formation of angiotensin, a chemical in the body that causes blood vessels to tighten, thus causing the vessels to relax. Because they are eliminated from the body by both the liver and the kidneys, they are safer to use in people with chronic kidney problems than drugs excreted by the kidneys alone. Common ACE inhibitors are lisinopril (*Prinivil, Zestril*), captopril (*Capotin*), and enalapril (*Vasotec*). Lisinopril has become extremely popular—it was the second most frequently prescribed generic drug in 2014 with more than 100 million prescriptions.

ACE inhibitors can cause birth defects and should not be taken during pregnancy. The most common side effect of ACE inhibitors is a chronic dry, hacking cough that occurs in up to 25 percent of people who take them. They can also cause a dangerous increase in the potassium level of the blood when taken with other medications that affect potassium. Other side effects include headache, dizziness, problems with erections, fatigue, and skin rash. Taking nonsteroidal anti-inflammatory pain relievers such as aspirin, ibuprofen, and naproxen can decrease the effectiveness of ACE inhibitors.

Angiotensin II Receptor Blockers (ARBs)

ARBs act similarly to ACE inhibitors, blocking the effects of angiotensin on blood vessels, causing them to relax. They are often prescribed to people who have problems taking ACE inhibitors, since they are less likely to cause a chronic cough. Otherwise, their side effects are similar to those of the ACE inhibitors—headaches, dizziness, increased potassium levels, sexual dysfunction, and skin rash. Common ARBs are losartan (*Cozaar*), valsartan (*Diovan*), and olmesartan (*Benicar*).

Calcium Channel Blockers (CCBs)

Calcium channel blockers interfere with the passage of calcium through cells, causing blood vessels to relax. Some of them also slow down the heart. Common CCBs include amlodipine (*Norvasc*), diltiazem (*Cardizem*), and nifedipine (*Procardia*). Calcium channel blockers, as well as thiazide diuretics, are more effective in lowering blood pressure in African Americans than beta-blockers, ACE inhibitors, and ARBs. This has been reported in several studies but the reason is unclear.

Constipation and headaches are the most common side effects of CCBs. Others include swollen ankles, dizziness, and skin rash. As with other high blood pressure medications, men can experience difficulties with erections. If you are taking a CCB, you should avoid grapefruit juice, which can increase the amount of CCB entering your bloodstream and could cause a dangerous drop in blood pressure.

Combination Therapy for Hypertension

If you are taking a blood pressure medication, you may have been prescribed one that is a combination of two, or in some cases three, different drugs. While some guidelines recommend sticking with one agent (monotherapy) at increasingly higher doses until blood pressure targets are met, many doctors start therapy with a low dose combination product, such as a diuretic with a beta-blocker or an

ACE inhibitor. Taking only one combination pill is easier for many people and the side effects of each component may be less at lower doses. *Lopressor HCT*, a combination of a thiazide diuretic and a beta-blocker, is a common combination. However, the safety of combining these different drugs long-term has not been established and additional research is underway.

Type of Blood Pressure Medication	Examples (Brand Name)	How They Work	Possible Side Effects
Thiazide diuretics	Hydrochlorothiazide (*Microzide*); Chlortalidone (*Thalitone*)	Cause the kidneys to eliminate larger amounts of sodium and water, decreasing blood volume and lowering the pressure inside the arteries	Frequent urination, erection problems, and potassium loss
Beta-blockers	Atenolol (*Tenormin*); Metoprolol (*Lopressor*); Propranolol (*Inderal*)	Block the hormones norepinephrine and epinephrine, causing the heart to beat less forcefully and dilating the blood vessels	Depression, insomnia, erection problems, constipation, diarrhea, nausea and vomiting, dizziness, fatigue, and cold hands and feet; asthma in people with lung disease

Angiotensin converting enzyme (ACE) inhibitors	Lisinopril (*Prinivil, Zestril*); Captopril (*Capoten*); Enalapril (*Vasotec*)	Block the formation of angiotensin, causing blood vessels to relax	Chronic dry, hacking cough, headache, dizziness, erection problems, fatigue, and skin rash; increased potassium levels when taken with certain other drugs
Angiotensin II receptor blockers (ARBs)	Losartan (*Cozaar*); Valsartan (*Diovan*); Olmesartan (*Benicar*)	Block the effects of angiotensin on blood vessels, causing them to relax	Headaches, dizziness, erection problems, fatigue, and skin rash; increased potassium levels when taken with certain other drugs
Calcium channel blockers (CCBs)	Amlodipine (*Norvasc*); Diltiazem (*Cardizem, Dilacor XR*); Nifedipine (*Adalat CC, Procardia*)	Interfere with the passage of calcium through cells, causing blood vessels to relax	Constipation, headaches, erection problems, swollen ankles, dizziness, and skin rash; avoid grapefruit juice—can cause a dangerous blood pressure drop

THE DANGERS OF LOW BLOOD PRESSURE

If you do take a drug for hypertension, it is important to monitor your blood pressure at least once a week to make sure it is not too low. There are dangers of having a blood pressure that is too low, especially in the elderly. Studies have confirmed that aggressive blood pressure treatment can lead to negative outcomes.

Cognitive Impairment (Poor Mental Functioning)

When I was a young family practice resident, the director of my program told us that the optimal systolic blood pressure was 100 plus a person's age. Dr. Auckerman said that as people age and their arteries harden, more force is needed to push blood into the brain. He was concerned that if blood pressure was too low, the brain would not get enough blood and the result would be a decline in mental functioning leading to dementia. While this advice is now considered outdated, there is growing evidence that when blood pressure is too low, poor mental functioning can occur.

Authors of a twelve-year study of more than 3,000 African Americans aged sixty-five or older reported that blood pressures below 120/70 were linked with cognitive impairment. They found that the best mental functioning was associated with a blood pressure of approximately 135/80. In another study of patients who already had dementia or mild cognitive impairment, those taking high blood pressure medication and had systolic pressures less than 128 mm Hg had a significantly greater mental decline over a nine month period. These studies both suggest that excessive blood pressure lowering may be harmful for older patients, especially those with cognitive problems.

Conversely, older people with blood pressures that are higher than the guidelines recommend have been found to have fewer problems with mental functioning. In an Italian study of people aged seventy-five or older, those who had systolic blood pressures that averaged 170 mm Hg had better scores on a mental status exam than those in the groups with average systolic pressures of 130 and 140. Perhaps Dr. Auckerman was not so far off base with his 100-plus-your-age theory.

Injuries from Falling

Hypertension medications can cause dizziness and a sudden drop in blood pressure when standing up too fast, increasing the risk of falls, broken hips, and head injuries. A study that followed nearly 5,000 adults over age seventy for three years reported that those taking high blood pressure medicines were 28 to 40 percent more likely to have a serious fall injury—broken bones, head trauma, or dislocated joints—than those not taking medication. Those who had suffered a fall injury in the past were more than twice as likely to have another one if they were on hypertension drugs.

Risk of Dying

People with blood pressure that is too low also have a higher risk of dying. In a study of more than 14,000 veterans ages forty-five to eighty-five, those with a diastolic blood pressure less than 70 mm Hg had a 50 percent increased risk of dying during the two years of the study. Another study of frail nursing home residents found that those with a systolic blood pressure less than 130 mm Hg who were taking two or more blood pressure medications had twice the risk of dying in the next two years compared to those taking less than two. Interestingly, those with systolic pressures less than 130 who were not taking hypertension drugs did not have this increased risk. Both of these studies make me question whether official guidelines place too much emphasis on blood pressure that is too high and not enough on the ill effects of blood pressure that is too low.

WHAT IS THE OPTIMAL BLOOD PRESSURE?

Two reports that were published in late 2015 with much media fanfare are being used to encourage doctors to treat high blood pressure more aggressively. They reported better outcomes in patients who were treated to a systolic blood pressure below 120 or 130 mm Hg. When I looked at these studies, however, I was not impressed. Both studies required participants to take a large number of drugs, the results were only minimally significant, and the incidence of side effects was concerning.

In the first, a review of nineteen different studies, intensive blood pressure lowering reduced strokes and heart attacks by modest amounts but had no impact on heart failure, deaths from heart disease, total deaths, or end-stage kidney disease. It was reported that 24.3 percent of the patients in the intensive therapy group used four or more antihypertensive drugs and 31.8 percent used three drugs. Only six of the nineteen studies reported on side effects and of these, there was a nearly threefold increase in serious episodes of low blood pressure.

The other report was of the SPRINT study, in which more than 9,000 people at a high risk of heart disease were randomized to receive medications to keep their systolic blood pressure either below 140 mm Hg (low intensive) or below 120 mm Hg (high intensive). The study was stopped after three years because the results supposedly showed better outcomes in the high intensive treatment group. In fact, the difference in outcomes between the two groups was very small—less than 1 percent. A bad outcome—heart attack, stroke, heart failure, or death from heart disease—occurred in 2.19 percent of those in the group whose systolic pressure was kept below 140 compared to a bad outcome of 1.65 percent in the group treated to a systolic of less than 120.

The researchers calculated that sixty-one people would need to be treated with the high intensive program in order to prevent one bad outcome and 172 to prevent a death from heart disease. In the meantime, those in the high intensive therapy group, who took an average of 2.8 medications compared with 1.8 for the others, had more than three times the incidence of kidney damage. Serious adverse events related to treatment, such as syncope—fainting from low blood pressure—were more than twice as common in the high intensive group. Mental functioning was not evaluated in the study nor was the incidence of broken bones or head trauma from falls.

A much larger study analyzed records from nearly 400,000 members of a large health maintenance organization who were taking high blood pressure medication. People who had blood pressures of 130 to 139 systolic and 60 to 79 diastolic were less likely to die or experience kidney failure than those either above or below those levels. Those with a systolic pressure of 110 to 119 had nearly twice the incidence of death and kidney failure, while those with a pressure below 110 had four times the risk of these events. On the other hand, a systolic pressure of 150 or above increased the risk of death and kidney failure.

DO YOU REALLY NEED THAT BLOOD PRESSURE PILL?

The first step is to find out if you really have high blood pressure. Don't let just one value at the doctor's office determine your diagnosis of hypertension. Check your blood pressure twice a day for a week to see what your resting values really are. After that, your options depend on what readings you find.

Blood Pressure 120–140/80–90 (Pre-hypertension)

Consider this a wake-up call and get busy exercising and making the changes in your diet that can lower your blood pressure and prevent it from going higher.

Blood Pressure 140–160/90–100 (Mild Hypertension)

You face a more difficult choice. Many doctors will want to start you on blood pressure medication right away, but you might be able to convince yours to wait. You don't want to go through life with your blood pressure this high, but trying lifestyle changes for a few months might be worthwhile. Studies confirm that a combination of a healthy diet, salt restriction, and exercise can reduce your blood pressure enough to take you out of the mild hypertension category. If you don't want to try lifestyle changes, or if they don't work for you, then taking medication to reduce your blood pressure to below 140/90, or below 150/90 if you are older than sixty, will lessen your risk of developing heart disease.

Blood Pressure More than 160/100 (Moderate to Severe Hypertension)

You need to start medication right away to bring down your blood pressure to an acceptable level. Lifestyle changes are still important, though, and may reduce the amount of medicine you will need to take. A healthy lifestyle will also reduce your overall chances of developing heart disease, as well as other chronic diseases such as diabetes.

Having a diagnosis of hypertension can be scary. Fortunately, there are many things you can do to decrease your risk of heart disease. Healthy lifestyle choices along with self-monitoring of blood pressure can help you to eliminate or reduce your need to take that pill.

IF YOU DO TAKE MEDICATION FOR HIGH BLOOD PRESSURE

- Monitor your blood pressure regularly to make sure it doesn't get too low.
- Be alert for orthostatic hypotension—dizziness that occurs when you stand up suddenly after sitting or on rising from bed.
- If you think you are having a side effect, let your doctor know right away. It is possible that a different medicine might be better for you.
- As with other drugs, be careful about taking medicines that have been on the market for only a short time. Their long-term side effects might not become evident for five to ten years.
- Ask your pharmacist or consult a website like www .drugs.com to make sure that there are not any dangerous interactions with other medications you are taking.

Chapter 9

Type 2 Diabetes

A ccording to official government reports, there are more than 30 million people in the United States with diabetes, or 9.4 percent of the total population. In those aged sixty-five or older, more than one out of four are said to have diabetes. The CDC estimates that more than seven million people with diabetes do not know that they have it. Clearly, diabetes is a huge public health problem.

WHAT IS DIABETES?

Diabetes occurs when there is a problem with how the body produces or responds to the hormone insulin. If there is not enough insulin, glucose—the most simple type of sugar—will not get into the cells. In type 1 diabetes, also called "juvenile-onset," the cells in the pancreas that produce insulin are inactive. Glucose builds up in the blood and urine, leading to weight loss, fatigue, increased thirst, and increased urination. If left untreated, this can lead to serious illness and even death. Treatment with insulin allows people with type 1 diabetes to lead healthy and productive lives.

Type 2 Diabetes

The good news is that only 5 to 10 percent of people with diabetes have type 1. The rest have type 2, also known as "adult-onset diabetes." In this disorder, the pancreas still produces insulin but it either doesn't produce enough or the body doesn't respond appropriately to it. Glucose builds up in the bloodstream instead of going into the cells. Symptoms, which are similar to those in type 1, can be mild and it can take years for someone to realize they have this problem.

Often, type 2 diabetes is discovered after a routine battery of laboratory tests. These tests include the fasting blood sugar (FBS) test, administered first thing in the morning after not eating for at least eight hours, and the glucose tolerance test (GTT), which measures blood sugar two hours after drinking a standardized dose of glucose. Both of these tests offer a snapshot of a certain moment in time, but may not reflect a person's overall range of blood glucose levels. They should be measured more than once to get an accurate result.

A better test is the hemoglobin A1c (HbA1c) test, which measures the percentage of blood sugar attached to a protein (hemoglobin) in red blood cells. The A1c level is an indication of the average glucose level in your blood over the previous two to three months. A diagnosis of type 2 diabetes is made with one or more of the following:

- Fasting blood sugar greater than 125
- Glucose tolerance test 200 or more
- HbA1c over 7.0 percent

Prediabetes

More disturbing is the number of people with what is called "prediabetes." More than a third of all adults aged eighteen or older (more than 84 million people), including almost half of those six-ty-five and older, are said to have this disorder. Prediabetes is a relatively new diagnosis that is based on abnormal laboratory tests alone:

- Fasting blood sugar between 100 and 125
- Glucose tolerance test between 140 and 199
- HbA1c of 5.6 to 6.9 percent

If you have been diagnosed with prediabetes, don't worry—it doesn't necessarily mean you will get diabetes. In fact, having a diagnosis of prediabetes can be seen as a wake-up call. It is not too late for you to make healthy lifestyle changes that will keep you from progressing to type 2 diabetes.

There is controversy about testing for abnormal glucose levels in healthy people, since giving someone a medical diagnosis such as prediabetes can create anxiety. However, lifestyle interventions such as a healthy diet and physical activity have been shown in several studies to reduce the likelihood of prediabetes progressing to type 2. Without healthy lifestyle changes 15 to 30 percent of people with prediabetes will develop type 2 diabetes within five years. Current recommendations are to test for abnormal blood glucose in people who are over age forty and are overweight, as well as those under age forty with risk factors such as obesity, high blood pressure, or high cholesterol.

Risk Factors for Developing Diabetes

There are several risk factors for developing type 2 diabetes. These include obesity (a body mass index of more than 30), a family history of diabetes, Asian ethnic group, hypertension, and ele-vated triglyceride levels. There are several medications for heart disease—statins, niacin, thiazide diuretics, and beta-blockers—that can increase the risk of developing diabetes by 9 to 43 percent. On the other hand, lifestyle interventions involving diet and exercise can reduce the risk of developing diabetes by up to 50 percent.

MANAGING TYPE 2 DIABETES WITHOUT DRUGS

There is no doubt that people with type 1 diabetes should take insulin. But if you have prediabetes or type 2, the first and foremost thing to do, recommended by the Mayo Clinic and other expert groups, is to make changes in your lifestyle that will help keep your blood sugar under control. In fact, many people can successfully manage their type 2 diabetes without drugs by losing weight, eating a healthy diet, exercising, and becoming educated about monitoring their blood sugar. In an analysis that combined the results from sixteen different studies, researchers found that patients who made lifestyle changes were able to reduce their A1c levels significantly, as well as their weight and blood pressure.

Weight Loss

Diabetes goes hand in hand with obesity. As the number of people with obesity has grown—now one-third of all Americans—so has the incidence of type 2 diabetes. Some people who are obese have a double problem with insulin—their body makes less of it and their cells do not respond to it as they should. This causes their blood glucose to become elevated. Not all obese people develop diabetes. Those with fat that accumulates around the abdomen—the so-called "apple shape"—seem to be at more risk of diabetes than those with fat in other areas.

The good news is that even a moderate weight loss of 5 to 10 percent of body weight can reduce A1c and other blood glucose levels significantly. For someone weighing 200 pounds, this mean losing ten to twenty pounds. A person who weighs 150 would have to lose seven to fifteen pounds. Not easy, but doable for most of us. Another benefit of such a weight loss—blood pressure and HDL cholesterol also will improve. And those losing 10 to 15 percent of body weight have even more of these health benefits.

Healthy Eating

There is no specific diet for diabetes but, as for many other diseases, eating healthy foods such as fresh fruits and vegetables, nuts, and whole grains is recommended. The Mediterranean diet includes all of these and has been found to help people with type 2 diabetes manage their illness without drugs. In a study conducted in Italy, overweight patients with type 2 diabetes were randomly assigned to either a Mediterranean diet (MD) or a low-fat (LF) diet. After four years, those in the MD group had better control of blood sugar and were less likely to need drugs than those following the LF diet.

People with diabetes also should cut down on eating sweets and refined carbohydrates, if not eliminate them altogether. The emphasis on low-fat diets over the past few decades caused people to eat more of these unhealthy carbohydrates, contributing to the current epidemics of type 2 diabetes and obesity. White bread, white rice, and white pasta, along with foods and beverages containing sugar, have what is known as a *high glycemic index*. This means that they cause a rapid increase of blood sugar, contributing to the development of diabetes.

White potatoes also have a high glycemic index. A study that analyzed data from nearly 200,000 healthy adults who were followed for up to twenty-four years found that eating potatoes increased the risk of developing type 2 diabetes. People who ate seven or more servings a week of potatoes had a 33 percent increased risk of diabetes compared to those who ate only one serving. French fries were the worst form of potatoes for diabetes risk when compared with baked, boiled, or mashed potatoes. Researchers also estimated that replacing three servings a week of potatoes with whole grains could reduce the risk of diabetes by 12 percent.

Other studies have linked the development of diabetes with sugary soft drinks, as well as sweetened milk drinks like milk shakes or flavored milk. Replacing the daily consumption of one serving of a sugary drink with either water or unsweetened tea or coffee can lower the risk of developing type 2 diabetes by 14 to 25 percent. And in an alarming study published in 2015, sugary beverages were blamed for causing an estimated 130,000 diabetes deaths worldwide each year.

Exercise

Regular physical activity has long been known to reduce or eliminate the need for diabetes medication. Besides the obvious benefit of weight loss, exercise makes insulin more effective in moving glucose from the bloodstream into the body's cells.

Physical activity and modest weight loss can lower type 2 diabetes risk by up to 58 percent in high-risk populations, including those with prediabetes. In a joint position statement, the American College of Sports Medicine and the American Diabetes Association stated: "Diet and PA (physical activity) are central to the management and prevention of type 2 diabetes. . . . When medications are used to control type

2 diabetes, they should augment lifestyle improvements, not replace them."

Studies suggest that a combination of aerobic exercise and strength training is best for controlling blood sugar. Moderate exercise such as walking, biking, or dancing for thirty minutes at least five days a week is recommended along with resistance activities such as weight lifting, yoga, and Pilates. Establishing a regular routine for exercise is important to make sure it becomes a part of your daily regimen. Before starting to exercise, make sure to get the okay from your doctor.

Judy, a fifty-five-year-old administrator for a nonprofit organization, had been putting on weight since her last child was born. While she gained only about two pounds a year, after twenty years it added up to forty extra pounds. Her sedentary job didn't help much. She was working full-time while raising a family and had little time for exercise. When she started feeling run-down, she visited her doctor. A routine battery of tests revealed an A1c level of 7.5, which led her doctor to diagnose type 2 diabetes.

When her doctor said that she needed to start taking medication, Judy balked. She asked if there was something else she could do instead. She had a bad reaction to penicillin when she was in college and didn't like taking pills. Her doctor suggested that she try changing her diet and getting more exercise to see if she could lower her A1c level without medication.

Judy was highly motivated to stay off drugs, so she got to work making changes in her life. She cut out processed foods and refined sugars and increased her intake of fruits and vegetables to five servings a day. She joined a gym and started taking Zumba classes three times a week. After a month she had lost ten pounds, which gave her the confidence to continue with her new habits.

When she returned to her doctor after six months, she had lost thirty pounds. Her A1c was down to 6.5 percent and her other glucose values were normal.

Three years later, Judy continues to enjoy a healthy lifestyle. She is taking classes to become a certified Zumba instructor and volunteers in a diabetes prevention program. She tells everyone that owing to healthy lifestyle changes, she feels at least ten years younger.

MEDICATIONS FOR TYPE 2 DIABETES

If making lifestyle changes is not enough to control your blood sugar, you may need to take medication. As with all drugs, you should weigh their benefits against the risks of short- and long-term dangers. Most people with type 2 diabetes can do well with oral medications but a small minority need to take insulin. The medications long used for this illness—metformin and the sulfonylureas—are now available as inexpensive generic formulations.

Metformin

Metformin, with trade names such as *Glucophage* and *Glumetza*, is recommended as the first choice for treatment of type 2 diabetes by physician groups in both the United States and Europe. It acts by reducing the amount of glucose produced by the liver as well as increasing the sensitivity of cells to insulin so that more glucose can be absorbed. Metformin can cause weight loss and reduces heart attacks and overall deaths compared to other diabetes medications.

Metformin has a very good safety record and for most people with type 2 diabetes, lifestyle changes along with metformin are enough to keep their A1c levels less than 7. If, after three to six months, these values do not come down to an acceptable level, a second drug is usually added.

Metformin Side Effects

The most common side effects of metformin are gastrointestinal, including nausea, vomiting, flatulence, and diarrhea. These can be lessened by taking it with meals and the side effects often go away over time. A serious side effect of metformin is lactic acidosis, a metabolic disorder caused by lack of oxygen in cells and the buildup of acid in the blood. Symptoms of this include fatigue, muscle pain, drowsiness, and difficulty breathing. Lactic acidosis is very rare and mostly occurs in people who already have kidney or liver disease. It can also occur from drinking too much alcohol while on metformin.

Sulfonylureas

These drugs, which include *Diabinese*, glyburide, and glipizide, are among the most commonly prescribed for type 2 diabetes after metformin. They act by stimulating the pancreas to secrete more insulin, lowering blood sugar. Because they are inexpensive and have an established track record, they are sometimes used as first-line treatment or in combination with metformin. However, more and more evidence is accumulating about their adverse effects and some experts recommend against taking them at all.

Sulfonylureas Side Effects

People sometimes gain five to eight pounds in the first year of treatment with sulfonylureas. The biggest danger with sulfonylureas, however, is hypoglycemia, or low blood sugar. This happens in up to 10 percent of people taking them, much more frequently than with other oral diabetes drugs.

Hypoglycemia can happen suddenly and is usually mild, causing shakiness and light-headedness. If left untreated, however, hypoglycemia can get worse and cause confusion, clumsiness, or fainting. Severe hypoglycemia can lead to seizures, coma, and even death. People taking sulfonylureas have two and a half times the risk of hypoglycemia than those taking metformin. Sulfonylureas also are more likely than other oral agents to cause hypoglycemia when prescribed in combination with metformin.

There is evidence that treatment with sulfonylureas leads to an increased risk of death. Researchers who analyzed data on patients with type 2 diabetes in the United Kingdom found one and a half times the number of deaths from all causes in those taking sulfonylureas compared with metformin users. This could be due to reports of an increased cancer risk, as well as an increased risk of heart disease with sulfonylureas.

Close monitoring of blood sugar when taking a sulfonylurea can help to prevent hypoglycemia. Home glucose testing with blood from a finger prick and an inexpensive electronic device allows people to monitor their blood glucose values and helps prevent the consequences of very high or very low blood sugar.

John first found out that he had type 2 diabetes after visiting his doctor because he was feeling stressed. It had been a difficult year for him as a small business owner, with sales down and rising costs. He had put on weight and was eating fast food more often than he liked. He and his doctor were both surprised when his fasting blood sugar results came back from the lab at 384 and his A1c was 12.8 percent. He started taking metformin right away and his A1c went down to the low 6s in four to five months.

John checks his blood sugar regularly at home. His doctor told him that if it got close to 200, he should take a low dose of glyburide, a sulfonylurea. When he tried this the first time, his blood sugar dropped one hundred points in an hour and he began feeling sweaty and jittery. Fortunately, he recognized the symptoms of hypoglycemia and drank a glass of orange juice, which evened things out. Now when his blood sugar gets too high, he takes only one-fourth of a glyburide, which brings it down about fifty points. He always carries a candy bar or sugary drink in his car in case he feels hypoglycemic.

John has improved his diet but still doesn't get enough exercise and is overweight. He is looking forward to retirement, when he will have time to go to the gym and get back in shape. He has noticed that when he is more physically active, his blood sugar is much easier to control. He hopes that once he starts a regular exercise program, he won't have to take the glyburide at all.

Other Medications for Type 2 Diabetes

There has been an explosion of new drugs for type 2 diabetes in the past ten years. This is likely due to the alarming number of people being diagnosed with this disorder, as well as the desire of the pharmaceutical industry to find new ways to profit. Given the more than 30 million people in the United States with diabetes, the market is huge and the pharmaceutical industry has responded with as many as twelve new types of drugs. Two out of the top-ten-selling brand-name drugs for the year ending in June 2015, *Lantus* and *Januvia*, were new diabetes medications.

The average price of one of these new drugs, a DPP-4 inhibitor, was $8.92 per pill in 2013 compared with $0.31 per pill for generic metformin. Whereas a month's supply of a generic sulfonylurea might cost $15, many of these newer drugs top $300 per month. In poor countries or for people without good health insurance, they are not a realistic option.

Dipeptidyl Peptidase-4 (DPP-4) Inhibitors

These drugs, which include sitagliptin (*Januvia*), saxagliptin (*Onglyza*) and linagliptin (*Tradjenta*), block an enzyme that reduces the production of insulin. They are sometimes recommended as the next line of therapy if metformin alone is not enough to lower blood sugar. They do not cause weight gain and the risk of hypoglycemia is low. They can lower A1c by 0.5 to 1 percent, which is comparable to sulfonylureas. *Januvia*, manufactured by Merck, was the eighth most prescribed drug in the twelve-month period ending in June 2015, with sales of $3.8 billion.

The FDA recently issued a safety announcement that DPP-4 inhibitors can cause severe and disabling joint pain. Some patients developed pain after taking them for just one day while it took several years for pain to occur in others. Symptoms usually went away within a month of stopping the medication. There have also been indications that DPP-4 inhibitors can increase the risks for heart failure, acute pancreatitis, mouth ulcers, and kidney failure. Because these drugs have been on the market for less than ten years, their long-term effects are unknown.

Glucagon-like Peptide-1 (GLP-1) Receptor Agonists

Exenatide (*Byetta*) and liraglutide (*Victoza*) are examples of GLP-1 receptor agonists. These injectable medications lower blood sugar by mimicking a hormone, glucagon, that stimulates the release of insulin. They also slow down digestion, causing decreased appetite and thus weight loss in some people. The risk of hypoglycemia is low with these agents, making them an attractive choice for blood sugar control. One downside of GLP-1 agonists is that they require daily or weekly shots, depending on the medication. Their cost also is more than $300 per month.

The most common side effects of GLP-1 agonists are nausea and vomiting, which are said to go away after the early days of treatment. Along with DPP-4 inhibitors, these medications have been associated with acute pancreatitis. In a study of diabetic patients, those who had taken a GLP-1 agonist in the past thirty days had more than twice the odds of being hospitalized for acute pancreatitis than nonusers. The FDA issued a communication in 2013 that it was evaluating these reports about pancreatitis but has not issued its final conclusions.

Sodium-glucose Co-transporter 2 (SGLT2) Inhibitors

These include canagliflozin (*Invokana*) and dapagliflozin (*Farxiga*), among others. They lower blood sugar by causing the kidneys to excrete glucose into the urine, rather than absorbing it back into the bloodstream. They are the new kids on the block among diabetes drugs, so evidence of adverse effects is just now emerging. A month's supply can cost upward of $300.

The most common side effects from SGLT2 inhibitors are yeast and urinary tract infections, both due to the heavy dose of sugar in the urine of people who take them. Two other more serious side effects of these drugs have been identified—ketoacidosis, a condition of too much acid in the blood, and bone fractures.

In 2015, the FDA issued safety announcements about the risk of ketoacidosis from SGLT2 inhibitors and required companies to include warnings on the labels of these medications. This was after twenty cases of patients requiring hospitalization were reported to the FDA in a little over a year. The announcements warned that "Patients should . . . seek medical attention immediately if they experience symptoms such as difficulty breathing, nausea, vomiting, abdominal pain, confusion, and unusual fatigue or sleepiness."

There was another FDA safety announcement in 2015 about the possibility of bone fractures and decreased bone density with these drugs. SGLT2 inhibitors can cause dizziness, which increases the chance of falls, and can increase phosphate levels in the blood, making bones more likely to break. People with risk factors for recurrent falls, such as the elderly, those with limited mobility, or those taking drugs that cause low blood pressure should avoid these agents. Yet another warning was issued by the FDA in May 2017, this time confirming an increased risk of leg and foot amputations with canagliflozin *(Invokana)*.

Two other possible long-term side effects of SGLT2 inhibitors have recently been added to the FDA watch list—an increased risk of strokes and blood clots and kidney injury. The watch list is a report of adverse events to alert physicians and patients that regulators have questions about a drug. Being on the watch list does not mean that there is a definite cause and effect, only that people should be aware of this possibility and watch out for it.

Thiazolidinediones

Rosiglitazone *(Avandia)* and pioglitazone *(Actos)* are examples of this class of drug. They cause the body to produce new cells that are more sensitive to insulin, allowing more glucose to get into them and lowering glucose levels in the blood. While these are some of the most efficient medications at lowering blood sugar, they have been associated with several problematic side effects and are no longer prescribed by many doctors.

Avandia was pulled off the market in 2010 after it was linked to tens of thousands of heart attacks, strokes, and heart failures. Its manufacturers were assessed $3 billion in 2012 after being found guilty of federal charges of a cover-up. It is now available only by special prescription for people who do not respond to other medications.

Actos is still available, but it can cause weight gain, swelling of extremities, and bone fractures. There is also evidence that *Actos* is associated with an increased risk of bladder cancer, especially in people taking it for more than two years. An analysis of nearly 146,000 patients found a 63 percent increased risk of bladder cancer in those taking *Actos*. In a disturbing development, low-dose *Actos* is now being promoted as a preventive treatment for people with prediabetes.

Injectable Insulin

You might wonder about the use of insulin, since it is mostly associated with type 1 diabetes. For some patients with type 2 diabetes, nightly insulin injections are preferable to an expensive medication with risky side effects. Since many of the oral drugs act by altering the production or sensitivity to insulin, supplying extra insulin itself can be a simpler way to reduce blood sugar. There are many newly patented insulin preparations on the market, including *Lantus* (insulin glargine), number five in top-selling drugs in the United States in 2015 with $5 billion in sales for the year. However, there is little evidence that this form of insulin is any better than NPH insulin, an intermediate acting one which has been used successfully for many years. The main danger of insulin is low blood sugar.

Type of Diabetes Medication	Examples (Brand Name)	How They Work	Possible Side Effects
Metformin	(*Glucophage*); (*Glumetza*); (*Fortamet*)	Reduce the amount of glucose produced by the liver as well as make body tissues more sensitive to insulin	Nausea, vomiting, flatulence, and diarrhea. Rarely lactic acidosis—fatigue, muscle pain, drowsiness, and difficulty breathing
Sulfonylureas	Chlorpropamide (*Diabinese*); Glyburide (*Micronase, DiaBeta*); Glipizide (*Glucotrol*)	Stimulate the cells of the pancreas to secrete more insulin	Low blood sugar, bloating, nausea, heartburn, anemia, and weight gain
DPP-4 inhibitors	Sitagliptin (*Januvia*); Saxagliptin (*Onglyza*); Linagliptin (*Tradjenta*)	Block an enzyme that reduces the production of insulin	Severe and disabling joint pain, acute pancreatitis, mouth ulcers, and heart and kidney failure

GLP-1 receptor agonists	Exenatide (*Byetta*); Liraglutide (*Victoza*)	Mimic the hormone glucagon that stimulates the release of insulin	Nausea, vomiting, and acute pancreatitis
SGLT2 inhibitors	Canagliflozin (*Invokana*); Dapagliflozin (*Farxiga*)	Cause the kidneys to excrete glucose into the urine	Yeast and urinary tract infections, ketoacidosis, dizziness, bone fractures, strokes and other blood clots, and kidney injury
Thiazolidinediones	Rosiglitazone (*Avandia*); Pioglitazone (*Actos*)	Cause the body to produce new cells which are more sensitive to insulin	*Avandia*—heart attacks, strokes, and heart failure *Actos*—weight gain, swelling of extremities, bone fractures, bladder cancer

ACCEPTABLE A1C LEVELS

Since A1c levels are now considered to be the gold standard for evaluating blood sugar control, you might ask—what is an acceptable level of A1c? For many years, the goal for all patients was to get below 7 percent. New guidelines, however, recommend a less stringent approach for people over age sixty, especially those who have long-standing diabetes, other chronic diseases, and are at greater risk for hypoglycemia. For this group, an A1c level of 7.1 to 8 is being proposed as a more reasonable target. This is based on studies that have shown that getting this group of patients below 7 percent was associated with increased hospitalizations, weight gain, severe hypoglycemia, and higher death rates.

Official Medication Guidelines

For those needing medication, there is widespread agreement that metformin should be the first one prescribed. In most cases, this drug along with diet and exercise will be enough to keep blood sugar within an acceptable range.

The official position of the American Diabetes Association, in a joint statement with its European counterpart, is that any one of five different types of drugs—sulfonylureas, thiazolidinediones, DPP-4 inhibitors, GLP1 agonists, or insulin—is acceptable to add to metformin if healthy eating, weight control, and exercise are not enough to control blood sugar. In practice, other factors such as cost and adverse effects should be taken into account on an individual basis when making a decision about medications.

Group Health Cooperative Guidelines

Group Health Cooperative, now part of Kaiser Permanente, is a large health maintenance organization in Washington State that has a conservative but sensible approach to the treatment of diabetes. New guidelines, issued to its medical practitioners in June 2015, recommend diet, exercise, and weight management as the backbone of diabetes care along with metformin if this is not enough to bring lab values within an acceptable range. They recommend that the A1c level be kept between 7 and 8 percent, with the caveat to "use clinical judgment to determine if a target lower than 7 percent is appropriate for an individual patient."

If A1c remains too high, the next step recommended is either a sulfonylurea drug or insulin. There are many newly patented insulin preparations on the market, including *Lantus* (insulin glargine), which, as mentioned before, was the fifth top-selling drug in 2015. The Group Health directive does not recommend *Lantus*, or other new patented insulin preparations, stating that these have no advantage over and are much more costly than regular NPH insulin. Most tellingly, Group Health specifically says it does *not recommend* any of the newer medications, including thiazolidine-diones, DPP-4 inhibitors, GLP1 agonists, and SGLT2 inhibitors.

DO YOU REALLY NEED THAT DIABETES DRUG?

The answer to this question depends on your individual situation. It is up to you and your physician to determine which of these drugs, if any, you need. Most experts recommend a stepwise approach to the management of type 2 diabetes. The first step for someone newly diagnosed, especially when their A1c level is below 8, is to make healthy lifestyle changes to see if that is enough to lower their blood glucose without medication. Keep in mind that diet, exercise, and weight control can be sufficient to reduce blood sugar for many people and that the long-term effects of many of the newer diabetes drugs are just now becoming evident.

If you need to take medication, diet and exercise can help reduce the amount you need. Once you are able to lower your A1c to an acceptable level, you might ask your doctor if a trial period without medication is possible. Finding a balance between blood sugar control and the risk of adverse side effects of medication should be your goal, as well as enjoying a healthy lifestyle.

As with many other diseases of our modern world resulting from the temptations of rich foods and sedentary hours in front of a screen, you can make the choice to change the habits that undermine your health, or you can take a pill.

Part Three

Safely Reducing Your Use of Drugs

Chapter 10

Talking to Your Doctor

It is important to have your doctor or health provider on board for any changes you make in your medications. But most of us are intimidated by the thought of questioning what our physician has prescribed. There is something about sitting in a small room clothed only in a flimsy gown with a fully dressed and authoritative doctor that makes us feel like five-year-olds. But take a deep breath, screw up your courage, and remember that it is *your* body and that this person is being paid by you or your health insurance company to serve you.

The good news is that many doctors are beginning to recognize the problem of polypharmacy and to discuss strategies for *deprescribing*—defined as "the process of tapering, withdrawing, discontinuing, or stopping medications." People aged sixty-five or older taking five or more prescription medications are more than twice as likely to have an adverse drug reaction than those taking only one or two. Approximately one out of five prescriptions for older adults is inappropriate. These findings are raising concern in the medical community. Millions of health-care dollars could be saved by reducing inappropriate medications and the costs associated with adverse side effects.

Experts are starting to question the practice of using multiple medications to drive down blood pressure, blood sugar, and cholesterol to levels recommended by official practice guidelines. Doctors are often rewarded financially to follow these guidelines, which are usually based on studies of people who have only one disease. These studies usually do not take into account other illnesses a person might have or interactions that might occur with the other drugs he is taking. And, as we learned in chapter 2, there are often financial relationships between those producing guidelines and the biomedical industry.

Following standardized guidelines often carries more risk of harm—falls, hospitalizations, and dementia—than good. Investigators reported that, if treated according to clinical practice guidelines, a hypothetical seventy-nine-year-old woman with five different illnesses would be prescribed nineteen doses of twelve different medications each day and be at risk for ten possible drug interactions.

BEFORE YOUR MEDICAL VISIT

There are several things that you can do in preparation for your next medical visit. Before you approach your doctor, be armed with the facts. When you make your appointment, let the office staff know that you want to discuss concerns about your medications and that you would like to be scheduled for some extra time.

Compile a Medication List

The first step in getting ready to talk to your doctor is to make a list of all the medications you are taking. This is especially important if more than one medical provider is prescribing drugs for you. This medication list should be printed and kept up-to-date. It should contain all of the following: name of the drug, strength of the drug, reason for taking it, and the dosage instructions. You can find this information on the labels of your medicine bottles. Make sure that you also include any vitamins or herbs you take. Here is an example based on some of the drugs my mother-in-law was taking.

SAMPLE MEDICATION LIST

Desipramine	10 mg	Depression	2 tablets at bedtime
Gabapentin	600 mg	Back pain	1 tablet three times a day
Lasix	40 mg	High blood pressure	1 tablet every morning
Amlodipine	10 mg	High blood pressure	1 tablet every morning
St. John's wort	300 mg	Depression	1 tablet three times a day
Vitamin D	800 IU	Bone health	1 tablet daily

It doesn't matter if you use the generic names or the brand names of the medications—your doctor will be familiar with both. Keep this list in your wallet or purse at all times and update it whenever something changes. Presenting this list to your doctor will let him know that you are serious about taking responsibility for your health and that you want to establish a collaborative relationship.

Check for Possible Interactions and Adverse Effects

Once you have this medication list, you can use the information to determine whether there are any potential drug-drug interactions or adverse side effects you might be having. Your doctor does not have time to do this in the short time allotted these days for medical visits. Look up your drugs on the Internet to see what side effects they can cause. Use the Drug Interactions Checker at www.drugs.com/drug_interactions.html to find out if any of your medications are likely to interact negatively with each other.

Be especially aware of drugs with dangerous side effects, such as anticholinergics, and those associated with serotonin syndrome (see chapter 1). After doing all of this, make a list of any questions or concerns that you have about a particular medication or combination of drugs.

Review the Relevant Chapters in This Book

If you are being treated for any of the illnesses covered in this book, consult that chapter to see if your blood values, blood pressure, or symptoms are in the category that absolutely needs to be treated with drugs, or if they are merely borderline. You can look up on the Internet some of the relevant studies listed in the back of this book that pertain to your problem. To find an abstract (summary) of a particular study, use a search engine such as Google to enter the name of the journal, date, volume, and page numbers of the reference—for example, *Health Aff.* 2016; 35:394–400—and a link will appear that you can use to go to the abstract. If you find a study that supports your desire to discontinue a specific drug, you can print it and show it to your doctor during your next visit.

AT YOUR MEDICAL VISIT

Most doctors do not like having their authority questioned, especially by their patients. You have to tread carefully in negotiating with them about your medications. Being patient, polite, and persistent is the key to bringing someone around to your way of thinking. Health providers do not have time at a typical office visit to go over all of your medications to determine which ones are really needed, especially when some of the drugs have been prescribed by specialists. So whatever groundwork you have done beforehand is especially valuable.

It is possible that your doctor is already aware of the need for deprescribing and will appreciate that you have taken the initiative to broach the subject. Introduce the topic early on in your visit, so that it is not left until the end when she is about to rush off. You could begin by asking her about your concerns—whether a medicine that you are taking is really needed or if you are taking too many different medicines. Show her your medication list and tell her if you are worried about any possible drug interactions or side effects.

At this point, your provider might try to reassure you that the drugs you are taking are safe and necessary and move on with the visit, but do not give up. Remember—it is *your* body. Let her know that you are willing to change your diet, to exercise, and to do some of the things that have been shown to be effective in treating your condition(s) without medications. This might be the moment to give her copies of any relevant studies. Tell her that you want to work with her to reduce your reliance on prescription drugs and that you hope she will support you in your efforts to do so.

You might be pleasantly surprised to find that your doctor is receptive to your request. She might be tired of handing out prescription after prescription but continues to do so because she thinks that's what people want. Finding someone who has made the effort to become informed about his health and the medications he is taking might feel like a breath of fresh air to her. On the other hand, a different doctor might feel insulted that you dare to question his judgement and become rude and dismissive of your concerns. If this happens, I recommend looking for another medical provider.

A supportive provider can help you decide which medications you really need and which ones are safe to discontinue. She can recommend which ones are safe to stop all at once and guide you in tapering off those that need to be discontinued more slowly. She, or her staff, might be able to refer you to local resources to support any lifestyle changes you plan to undertake or alternative therapies to explore.

HOW TO TALK TO YOUR DOCTOR

Before your visit:
- Prepare your medication list.
- Check your drugs for any possible adverse effects or drug interactions you might be having.

- Use the information in this book and your Internet search to determine which drugs you may not need.
- Compile a list of questions and concerns for your doctor about your medications.

At your visit:
- Introduce your questions and concerns early in the visit.
- Always be patient and polite, but also persistent.
- Remember that it is *your* body and that your provider is being paid to serve you.
- Let your doctor know that you want to work together as a team to reduce your reliance on prescription drugs.
- (Optional) Provide your doctor with copies of any studies that support your desire to discontinue a particular medication.

Chapter 11

Making Healthy Lifestyle Changes

Eighty percent of cardiovascular disease, the leading cause of death in the United States, could be prevented by changes in three lifestyle factors—diet, exercise, and smoking. But it takes effort to lead a healthy lifestyle in this day and age. Many of us spend hours at work in front of a computer. We come home tired and spend the evening in front of a screen, either scrolling on our phones through Facebook, turning on the television news, or binge-watching a series on Netflix. We are constantly bombarded by advertisements for unhealthy foods. Fast food outlets tempt us to grab a quick bite when we are out and about. It is hard to motivate ourselves to slice and dice the fruits and vegetables necessary for a healthy meal. We find it easier to pop a frozen pizza in the oven and call it dinner. Believe me, I know.

We drive everywhere—even when we are going only a short distance. If you live in a major urban center, you might be lucky enough to have public transportation a few blocks away. But most neighborhoods were not designed for walking, without sidewalks and safe places to cross the street. Our days are tightly scheduled, with little time to take a deep breath and relax. Even retirees have a jam-packed day filled with shopping, volunteer activities, hobbies, medical visits, and socializing with friends.

A recent survey found that only 2.7 percent of US adults met all four requirements for a healthy lifestyle—maintaining a healthy diet, exercising regularly, abstaining from smoking, and keeping their weight in check. Eleven percent met none of these criteria and 37 percent met at least two. The definitions for meeting these requirements were fairly stringent, but those who did had lower blood pressure, lower blood glucose, and lower LDL cholesterol levels than the others.

HEALTHY EATING

If you eat a diet composed mainly of fresh fruits and vegetables, whole grains, and fish, you will have a lower risk of developing the chronic diseases that we have covered in this book. On the other hand, eating large amounts of refined carbohydrates and added sugars will have a negative impact on your health. Let's review the evidence:

- Eating a Mediterranean diet—fish, fruits, vegetables, legumes, and olive oil—can reduce heart disease and deaths from all causes by as much as 30 percent, even in high-risk patients.
- The DASH diet—fruits, vegetables, whole grains, and low salt—lowered blood pressure by an average of 11.2 mm Hg systolic and 7.5 mm Hg diastolic in people with borderline or mild hypertension.
- Replacing one serving of a sugary drink each day with either water or unsweetened tea or coffee can lower the risk of developing diabetes by between 14 and 25 percent.

- Those who consume more refined carbohydrates and added sugars have an increased risk of depression, while those who eat more fiber, fruits, and vegetables have a lower risk.
- People following the Mediterranean diet have less than half the incidence of acid reflux as those on a diet of red meat, fried food, sweets, and junk food.

How to Change Your Eating Habits

You probably already know how important it is to eat healthy foods, but might find it difficult to incorporate a healthy eating plan into your life. Shopping for and preparing healthy meals takes time and effort, but the payoff is worth it.

Start with something small, like reducing your intake of red meat to once or twice a week and increasing the fish in your diet. Make an effort to eat five servings of fresh fruits and veggies each day, easier to do if half of your plate at each meal is covered by them. Switch from refined carbohydrates to whole-grain breads and pastas and substitute water for soft drinks and fruit for sugary desserts. Snack on nuts or dried fruit, rather than chips and cookies. Avoid eating processed foods and check labels when you are shopping to look for hidden sugar and salt. The website www .choosemyplate.gov/start-small-changes gives more specifics about healthy food choices.

In a hurry? Try adding leftover rotisserie chicken to a pre-packaged salad or keep canned beans on hand for a quick burrito on whole wheat tortillas. A stir-fry of tofu with chopped vegetables such as carrots, broccoli, and red peppers and a dash of soy sauce over brown rice is easy and filling. Try to eat things that you like and throw away any unhealthy foods that you have on hand. Eat slowly and savor each bite. Share meals with friends or family and do not eat in front of the television. For recipes and sample menus for healthy eating, see www.choosemyplate.gov /recipes-cookbooks-and-menus.

Eating at restaurants and at get-togethers with friends are the greatest challenges, since so many of our social activities are planned around food. If you are going to a potluck, take something healthy. At restaurants, choose foods that adhere to your diet plan, such as salads and grilled fish. Allow yourself to splurge once a week and eat something decadent—a rich pasta dish or a dessert. If you rein yourself in too tightly, you will likely fail. Make changes slowly and give yourself time to adjust to a new diet.

If you make these dietary changes, you will soon notice that you feel better, have more energy, and your outlook has improved. You will likely lose weight. What is more important—you will reduce your risk of many of the chronic diseases that plague our modern lives. At the same time, you will increase your chance of a long and healthy life. So what's stopping you?

EXERCISE

We all know that exercise is good for us and there is ample evidence that it can reduce the risk of many chronic diseases. Motivating ourselves to do it, however, can be difficult. If you are already exercising regularly, you can pat yourself on the back and skip the next few paragraphs. If not, here are some facts that may encourage you to start an exercise program:

- Physical activity and modest weight loss have been shown to lower type 2 diabetes risk by up to 58 percent in high-risk populations.

- Exercise is as effective as medication in treating depression and the results may be more long-lasting.
- Exercise has been found to reduce the risk of falling and subsequent hip fractures by as much as 60 percent.
- Moderate to vigorous physical activity three to four times a week decreases both systolic and diastolic blood pressure.
- A 64 percent increase in heart disease was found in men who reported twenty-four hours or more of sedentary activity per week.
- People living in walkable urban neighborhoods have a decreased risk of becoming overweight or of developing diabetes.
- Aerobic, strengthening, water, and tai chi exercises all improve pain and joint function in people with osteoarthritis of the hip or knee.

How to Get More Exercise

Experts agree that the best exercise is one that a person enjoys doing. If you like to dance, try Zumba or salsa lessons. If water is your thing, swimming or rowing are excellent choices. You can go to a gym to run on the treadmill or lift weights. Are you bookish? Going for long walks listening to audiobooks might be just the thing. If you are gregarious and outgoing, look into tennis or a team sport such as bowling. Think back to your childhood and try to remember what physical activities you enjoyed most. I recently heard about a tap dancing group for women over fifty that I might investigate. There is a whole world of possibilities out there for you to explore.

If you haven't exercised in a long time, start out slowly. Walking around the block once a day can be enough if you are seriously out of shape. Increase your distance every few days and before long you will begin to look forward to it. Exercise causes your body to produce endorphins, which will improve your mood. Having an exercise partner can help you keep up your routine. On a cloudy day when you hadn't slept well the night before, you might be tempted to skip a day if you aren't accountable to someone else.

The CDC recommends two kinds of exercise each week—aerobic and strength training. For optimum health, they recommend 150 minutes of moderate aerobic exercise each week, such as brisk walking, or 75 minutes a week of vigorous exercise, such as jogging or running. In addition, two or more days a week of muscle strengthening, such as lifting weights, is also recommended. Eighty percent of US adults do not meet this CDC exercise goal.

Some experts argue that these guidelines are too stringent and that encouraging people to have more modest exercise goals might be more realistic and attainable. One study found that in people aged sixty or older, those who exercised less than 150 minutes per week—on average 75 minutes—had a 22 percent decreased risk of death compared to people who were completely inactive. Other researchers have reported that replacing just two minutes of sitting every hour with light exercise, such as walking around, reduces the risk of death by one-third.

A seminar about obesity that I attended several years ago encouraged doctors to write out prescriptions for exercise and to hand them to patients. The speaker claimed that this was much more effective than a verbal recommendation. Here is my prescription for you for the *minimum* of exercise—walk briskly for at least 30 minutes three times a week.

SMOKING

The third lifestyle habit that is associated with increased death rates is smoking. This should come as no surprise, since we have known for a long while that it is associated with lung cancer and chronic obstructive pulmonary disease (COPD). Smoking also increases the risk of many other illnesses, including heart disease, osteoporosis, acid reflux, rheumatoid arthritis, and diabetes. The US Surgeon General's 2014 report on smoking contained the following facts:

- Nearly half a million Americans die prematurely from smoking each year.
- More than 16 million Americans suffer from a disease caused by smoking.
- Smoking causes 87 percent of lung cancer deaths, 32 percent of coronary heart disease deaths, and 79 percent of all cases of chronic obstructive pulmonary disease (COPD) in the United States.
- One out of three cancer deaths is caused by smoking.
- Cigarette smoking diminishes overall health status, impairs immune function, and reduces quality of life.

How to Stop Smoking

Fortunately, smoking is no longer as widespread as in past years, but 42 million American adults and about 3 million middle and high school students continue to smoke. If you are a smoker, it is never too late to quit. Long-term smokers aged sixty or above who quit smoking for at least five years were able to lower their risk of heart disease by one-third.

Ask your health provider about prescribing a nicotine patch or beginning a smoking cessation program. You can call

1-800-QUIT-NOW, the number operated by the National Cancer Institute (NCI), which will link you to your state's quitline. A related resource is www.smokefree.gov, which offers free web- and text-based programs to support your efforts to stop smoking. Don't be discouraged if you don't succeed on your first try. It often takes several efforts for people to quit completely.

WEIGHT REDUCTION

The fourth recommendation for healthy living is to keep your weight in check. Obesity is rampant in the United States—40 percent of women and 35 percent of men are obese, meaning they have a Body Mass Index (BMI) greater than 30. Another one-third are overweight, with a BMI between 25 and 30. Our culture and lifestyle are mostly to blame for this as we are surrounded by unhealthy foods and live mostly sedentary lives. (Check your BMI on www.bmi calculator.nct.)

We have seen in several chapters that losing just five to ten pounds can have a positive impact on many common chronic illnesses—diabetes, hypertension, osteoarthritis, acid reflux, and heart disease. Knowing that you need to lose weight is one thing. Actually losing it is more difficult.

How to Lose Weight

I am certainly no expert on losing weight and there are many bestsellers that will exhort you to follow a particular diet plan. Low-fat, low-carb, Atkins, paleo, grapefruit diet, vegan—I have seen many of them come and go over my lifetime and have tried my share of them. But I have come to believe that there is a simple formula for losing weight—burn more calories than you take in. Healthy eating and exercise are vitally important, but you won't lose weight unless your energy output is greater than your input.

In the osteoarthritis weight reduction program mentioned earlier, participants were limited to 1,200 calories each day and exercised for an hour three times a week. It took eighteen months, but the average weight loss was twenty pounds. This is an extreme diet and not necessary for most people, but it gives you an idea of what is possible. You can find an excellent resource to help determine the number of calories you need to eat each day, as well as how many you need to burn in order to lose weight, at www.cancer.org/healthy/toolsandcalculators/calculators/app /calorie-counter-calculator.

You can find calorie counters in handy paperbacks available at drugstores or on websites and in mobile apps. If you keep a food diary for a few days and also calculate how many calories you are burning through exercise and daily activities, you will have a good idea of what you need to do to lose weight. Many phone apps are now availabe to help you do this.

CHOOSING A HEALTHY LIFESTYLE

The benefits of choosing a healthy lifestyle cannot be overstated. Not only will you feel better, but you will lower your risk of many chronic diseases. In a landmark study entitled "Healthy living is the best revenge," researchers looked at the four healthy lifestyle factors we have covered in this chapter—eating a healthy diet of fruits, vegetables, and whole grains; performing three and a half hours of physical exercise each week; never smoking; and having a BMI of less than 30.

Only 9 percent of the more than 23,000 people in the study had all four healthy factors, but these people had a 93 percent lower risk of developing diabetes, 81 percent less risk of a heart attack, and were 50 percent less likely to have a stroke when compared to those with no healthy factors. Most people fell within the range of one to three healthy factors, and as the number of healthy factors increased, the risk of having a chronic disease decreased accordingly.

Do you *really* need that pill? Chances are that if you adopt healthy lifestyle practices, your need for pharmaceutical medications will drop dramatically. Even meeting the requirements for two or three healthy practices will improve your overall health and decrease your risk of a chronic disease. Go ahead—try it. You have nothing to lose except, perhaps, the number of pills you need to take.

Chapter 12

Alternative Therapies

If lifestyle modifications are not enough to bring your health problems under control, consider alternative therapies. As we have seen in several chapters, herbal remedies, such as St. John's wort for depression and supplements like glucosamine/chondroitin for osteoarthritis, are helpful in managing the symptoms of chronic illnesses. We've also seen evidence that acupuncture is effective in treating acid reflux, depression, back and knee pain, and high blood pressure. Published studies have shown improvements in depression and several types of pain with homeopathic medicines. Techniques that utilize the connection between the mind and the body—yoga, tai chi, cognitive behavioral therapy, and mindfulness meditation—are effective for chronic pain, depression, and high blood pressure, and can prevent cardiovascular disease and osteoporosis.

Some alternative treatments, such as supplements and herbs, act in ways that are similar to that of modern medicine, altering biochemical processes on the molecular level. Other modalities, such as acupuncture, naturopathy, and homeopathy, operate under a different paradigm of healing—that of stimulating the body's own self-healing mechanisms.

THE SELF-HEALING ABILITY OF OUR BODIES

The human body is a magnificently tuned orchestra, with many different parts that function harmoniously together. Its complex systems and feedback mechanisms are a marvel of efficiency and sophistication. Even the most advanced computer systems cannot rival the myriad and interconnected functions of the human organism.

Modern medicine has helped us to understand much about the underlying mechanisms of the human body. Each of its major systems—circulatory, digestive, endocrine, and so on—has been studied in exquisite detail and much is known about the biochemical pathways of its various processes. It is an organism that is built to last nearly a century, if all goes well. And many of the scourges of civilization—poor hygiene and sanitation, infectious diseases, and severe trauma—have been greatly reduced by advances in public health and modern medicine.

I once treated Joe, a professional hockey player, who had retired early due to osteoarthritis of the knee. It had all started with a collision on the ice that twisted his knee. The team doctor had given him a nonsteroidal anti-inflammatory drug to get him back into the game. The pain and swelling of the knee continued over the next few days, so Joe was given a shot of cortisone to enable him to finish the season. But he never fully recovered from the knee problem and developed osteoarthritis, which ultimately led to the end of his career at age twenty-five.

Chronic medical conditions, such as Joe's arthritis, have not been significantly improved by modern medicine. In fact, some illnesses, such as diabetes and cancer, are on the rise. Why is this happening, in spite of the many technological and scientific advances in medicine? I believe it is due to an important aspect of healing that has been lost in this last century of amazing medical progress—a respect for the self-healing capacity of the body. Modern medicine ignores the innate intelligence of the body that directs and manages its wondrous complexity. And it treats the body as if it were a machine that can be tinkered with in one area without a corresponding effect somewhere else.

Your Self-Healing Mechanisms at Work

If you look at your body's response to a cold virus, it is easy to see your self-healing mechanisms at work. The symptoms that you experience are not part of the disease itself; rather, they are part of your body's reaction to the illness, its attempt to fight off the cold. One of your first symptoms is sneezing—a forceful gust of air from the nose, which expels invading organisms. Coughing is another way your body tries to get rid of the virus. The mucus membranes lining your nose might start to secrete a watery fluid, another way to repel the attackers. Or your throat will become sore, as blood carrying white blood cells from the immune system rush to the scene to destroy and carry away the virus.

If the virus is a particularly nasty one, you will develop a fever, which increases the number of white blood cells the body produces to fight the infection. Your increased body temperature will prove deadly to some microorganisms. All of this happens without your conscious knowledge or volition. Your body's natural response is to protect you, to mount a strong defense when exposed to infectious agents such as viruses or bacteria.

What would happen if these defenses were immobilized? Consider a medieval town or castle, surrounded by a moat and then a high wall with archers positioned strategically on top. If you take away the archers, tear down the wall, and drain the moat, what will happen when an invading army comes through? The answer is obvious—it will march right into the town and take over. This is similar to what might happen when you take an over-the-counter medication to treat your cold symptoms. You will block your body's natural defenses and run a greater risk of a complication such as bronchitis or pneumonia.

Opposing the Body's Self-Healing Capacity

The medicines that you take for your cold actively work against the body's innate healing capacity, such as the antihistamine for your runny nose or the decongestant to open up your blocked nasal passages. Another example is the use of an antipyretic, such as aspirin or *Tylenol*, to bring down your fever. These medicines give you temporary relief but do nothing to help you fight the infection. In fact, they will do the opposite—immobilize your body's natural defense mechanisms and allow easier passage of the virus into your body.

Unfortunately, most of the drugs used in modern medicine today are based on this principle—to oppose or suppress the symptoms that the body is producing in its attempts to heal. While these drugs may relieve symptoms in the short term, they do nothing to support or enhance a person's overall health. And when such drugs are taken continuously and in combination with each other, the long-term effects cannot be beneficial.

Ignoring the wisdom of the body's inherent healing capacity will likely lead to worsened health. The human body is a dynamic, self-protecting, and self-healing system. If left alone, it usually will minimize the harmful results of illness and other stresses. But if it is constantly bombarded with drugs, these innate defenses will become weakened and ineffective.

This is what happened to the hockey player Joe. He should have stayed off his sprained knee, since the pain and swelling of the inflammatory response was a protective mechanism to force him to rest the injured part. Taking drugs to suppress his symptoms and continuing to play on the injury slowed the healing process and ultimately led to a career-ending chronic condition.

ALTERNATIVE HEALING SYSTEMS

Alternative healing systems recognize and promote the self-healing abilities of the body. This aspect of healing fell out of favor in the twentieth century, as modern medicine arrived with its dramatic surgeries and the promise of miraculous cures. But this concept needs to be incorporated into our modern understanding of health and disease if we are to comprehend the full impact of overmedication on the human body.

Acupuncture

Acupuncture is a five-thousand-year-old type of Chinese medicine that uses fine needles inserted in specific locations to remove blockages and regulate the flow of energy—called *chi*—in the body. It is based on the principles of *yin* and *yang*, which must be in proper balance for good health to occur. Most states require a diploma from the National Certification Commission for Acupuncture and Oriental Medicine for licensing. In looking for an acupuncturist, ask for recommendations from people who have had good results and make sure he is licensed to practice in your state.

Naturopathy

Naturopathy is based on the principle of *vis medicatrix naturae*—the healing power of nature. It is an eclectic brand of natural medicine that utilizes a wide variety of natural healing methods—herbal medicines, nutritional supplements, physical therapy, spinal manipulation, hydrotherapy, lifestyle counseling, homeopathy,

Chinese medicine, and detoxification. Naturopathic physicians have graduated from four-year naturopathic medical schools and are licensed to practice in many states. To find a naturopath near you, consult the American Association of Naturopathic Physicians' website, www.naturopathic.org.

Homeopathic Medicine

Homeopathy is based on the *principle of similars*, or like cures like. A substance that can cause symptoms in a healthy person is used to treat those same symptoms in someone who is sick. Homeopathic remedies are highly diluted preparations of natural substances that are given to stimulate the body's self-healing ability. They are used by many doctors in Europe, Latin America, and India. There is no formal licensing for homeopathy in the United States, but it is practiced by a variety of health practitioners, including naturopathic physicians and some medical doctors. The National Center for Homeopathy, www.homeopathycenter. org/, and the American Institute of Homeopathy, www.homeo pathyusa.org/, can provide information about homeopathic providers in your area.

A DELICATE BALANCE

There is a constant balancing act taking place within your body. On one side is the strength of your innate defense mechanisms; on the other, threats to your health, such as exposure to illness, external stress, or an inherited disease. To stay healthy and in balance, you need to maximize your defense mechanisms and minimize these harmful influences. Not everyone who is exposed to a cold virus gets sick—only those who are susceptible because their defenses are down, or those who inhale a particularly large dose of microorganisms.

Leading a healthy lifestyle is one way to optimize the self-healing capacity of your body—regular exercise, moderation in food and drink, adequate sleep, and avoidance of stress. But often that is not enough. We do not live in a perfect world and it is not possible to have a completely healthy lifestyle. Exposure to stress or disease can be so strong that it overwhelms the body's defense mechanisms. Fortunately, there are alternative treatments that can help restore health by strengthening the body's self-healing capacity.

The overuse of prescription drugs upsets the functioning of this highly sophisticated life system. How can we expect the body to respond favorably when it is inundated with several different foreign chemicals that not only have significant physiologic side effects but also block its internal protective mechanisms? We have seen in this book that dementia, chronic kidney disease, heart attacks, strokes, and bone fractures are some of the serious adverse effects of many commonly prescribed drugs. Rather than improving health, I am convinced that the overuse of multiple drugs is actually making people sicker.

Conclusion

There is no doubt that modern medicine has improved our lives in many ways. Without emergency surgery, I would have lost vision in my right eye after my retina detached ten years ago. My husband would not be alive today without open-heart surgery to replace his faulty aortic heart valve. I am extremely grateful for both of these things and know many people who have had similar benefits from advanced medical technology.

The advent of antibiotics has lessened the impact of many infectious diseases. And people with illnesses that in the past would have led to an early demise, such as cancer and HIV/AIDS, survive for many years after their diagnoses. We must not forget the contribution of epidemiology, which has helped us to understand the importance of clean air and water and the dangers of lead paint, pesticides, and cancer-causing chemicals in the environment. Vaccines have contributed to the near elimination of polio, smallpox, and tetanus. Laboratory scientists are probing deeper and deeper into the genetic causes of disease.

All of this has happened in a relatively short period of human history and yet, sometimes there is too much of a good thing. As you have learned from this book, the use of pharmaceutical drugs is out of control. Too many people are taking too many drugs that not only are unnecessary, but also are causing them more harm than good. The death rate in the United States increased in 2015, the first time since 2005, and remained the same in 2016. Surely, if taking five or more drugs were beneficial, we would see lower death rates, not rising ones. The biggest jump was in deaths from Alzheimer's disease. Mental impairment and dementia are associated with many of the most commonly used medications— statins, proton-pump inhibitors, antihistamines, tranquilizers, drugs for urinary incontinence, and certain antidepressants. Is it possible that the rise in Alzheimer's deaths is related to the overuse of these drugs?

I am hopeful that this epidemic of overmedication will subside as more and more people understand the ill effects of taking so many pharmaceutical drugs. There is no incentive for the drug industry to stop selling them, nor are there meaningful efforts within the medical profession to stop prescribing them. After reading this book, I hope that you are motivated to reduce or eliminate the use of the drugs that you don't really need, or those of a spouse, elderly parent, or grandparent about whom you are concerned. This book was written to help you decide—do you *really* need that pill?

Recommended Reading

John Abramson, *Overdosed America: The Broken Promise of American Medicine* (New York: HarperCollins Publishers, 2008).

Marcia Angell, *The Truth About the Drug Companies: How They Deceive Us and What to Do About It* (New York: Random House, 2005).

Shannon Brownlee, *Overtreated: Why Too Much Medicine Is Making Us Sicker and Poorer* (New York: Bloomsbury USA, 2007).

Ben Goldacre, *Bad Pharma: How Drug Companies Mislead Doctors and Harm Patients* (London: Faber and Faber, 2012).

David Healy, *Pharmageddon* (Berkeley: University of California Press, 2012).

Roy Moynihan and Alan Cassels, *Selling Sickness: How the World's Biggest Pharmaceutical Companies Are Turning Us All into Patients* (New York: Basic Books, 2005).

H. Gilbert Welch, *Less Medicine, More Health* (Boston: Beacon Press, 2015).

Chapter Source Notes

Introduction

xv **40 percent of people over age sixty-five regularly take five or more prescription drugs:** Centers for Disease Control and Prevention. Health United States 2011 with special feature on socioeconomic status and health. Accessed at: http://www.cdc.gov/nchs/data/hus/hus14.pdf#085, Table 85, pages 287–288.

xv **Study of recently hospitalized patients aged sixty-five:** Rohrer JE, Garrison G, Obehelman SA, et al. Epidemiology of polypharmacy among family medicine patients at hospital discharge. *J Prim Care Community Health*. 2013; 4: 101–105.

xv **One in five prescriptions for people in this age group:** Opondo D, Eslami S, Visscher S, et al. Inappropriateness of medication prescriptions to elderly patients in the primary care setting: a systematic review. *PLoS One*. 2012. https//doi.org/10.1371/journal.pone.0043617.

xv **21.8 percent of adults took three or more:** Centers for Disease Control and Prevention. Therapeutic Drug Use. May 14, 2015. Accessed at: http://www.cdc.gov/nchs/fastats/drug-use-therapeutic.htm.

xvi **The use of five or more drugs nearly doubled:** Trends in prescription drug use among adults in the United States from 1999–2012. *JAMA*. 2015; 314: 1818–1830.

xvi **Almost four hundred and fifty people in the United States die each day:** US Food and Drug Administration. FAERS Reporting System Public Dashboard. Accessed at: https://www.fda.gov/Drugs/Guidance

ComplianceRegulatoryInformation/Surveillance/AdverseDrugEffects
/ucm070093.htm

xvi **Those who took five or more drugs have nearly twice the risk:** Bourgeois
FT, Shannon MW, Valim C, et al. Adverse drug events in the outpatient
setting: an 11-year national analysis. *Pharmacoepidemiology and Drug
Safety.* 2010; 19: 901–910.

xvi **One-and-a-half million people in the United States are harmed each
year:** National Academies Institute of Medicine. Medication Errors Injure
1.5 Million People and Cost Billions of Dollars Annually. July 20, 2006.
Accessed at: http://www8.nationalacademies.org/onpinews/newsitem.
aspx?recordid=11623

xvi **Unintended drug overdoses, which first exceeded traffic accidents:**
Centers for Disease Control and Prevention. Drug Poisoning Deaths in
the United States, 1980–2008. NCHS Data Brief No. 81, December
2011.

xvii **In 2014, there were more than 47,000 accidental drug overdoses:** Rudd
RA, Aleshire N, JD1; Zibbell JE, et al. Increases in drug and opioid over-
dose deaths—United States, 2000–2014. *CDC Morbidity and Mortality
Weekly Report.* 2016; 64 (50); 1378–1382.

xvii **The number of drug overdose deaths reached 64,000:** National Institute
on Drug Abuse. Overdose death rates, September, 2017. Accessed at: https://
www.drugabuse.gov/related-topics/trends-statistics/overdose-death-rates

xvii **Misuse of nonsteroidal anti-inflammatory drugs:** Grissinger M. Top 10
adverse drug reactions and medication errors. Program and abstracts of the
American Pharmacists Association 2007 Annual Meeting, March 16–19,
Atlanta, Georgia; 2007.

xvii **The risk of falling is twice as likely:** Ziere G, Dieleman JP, Hofman A, et
al. Polypharmacy and falls in the middle age and elderly population. *Br J
Clin Pharmacol.* 2006; 61: 218–223.

xvii **Eight times more likely to suffer a hip fracture:** Lai SW, Liao KF, Liao
CC, et al. Polypharmacy correlates with increased risk for hip fracture in
the elderly: a population-based study. *Medicine.* 2010; 89: 295–299.

xvii **$380 billion in the United States in 2016:** Kaiser Family Foun-
dation. Total retail sales for prescription drugs filled at pharmacies,
2016. Accessed at: https://www.kff.org/health-costs/state-indicator/
total-sales-for-retail-rx-drugs/.

xvii Projected to reach $590 billion by 2020: IMS Health. Global Medicines Use in 2020: Outlook and Implications. November 12, 2015. Accessed at: https://www.imshealth.com/en/thought-leadership/ims-institute/reports /global-medicines-use-in-2020.

xvii Mayo Clinic study: Zhong W, Maradit-Kremers H, St. Sauver JL, et al. Age and sex patterns of drug prescribing in a defined American population. *Mayo Clin Proc.* 2013; 88: 697–707.

xvii More than $14 million a day were spent in 2015: Healthcare marketing. Advertising Age. October 17, 2016. Accessed at: http://gaia.adage.com /images /bin/pdf/KantarHCwhitepaper_complete.pdf

Chapter 1: The Dangers of Taking Too Many Pills

Adverse Side Effects

3 **106,000 people in the United States died annually:** Lazarou J, Pomeranz BH, Corey PN. Incidence of adverse drug reactions in hospitalized patients: a meta-analysis of prospective studies. *JAMA.*1998; 279: 1200–4.

4 **Number of reported deaths from ADRs reached more than 164,000 in 2017:** US Food and Drug Administration. FAERS Reporting System Public Dashboard. Accessed at: https://www.fda.gov/Drugs/GuidanceCompliance RegulatoryInformation/Surveillance/AdverseDrugEffects/ucm070093.htm.

4 **Tripled since 2006:** US Food and Drug Administration. Reports Received and Reports Entered into FAERS by Year. Accessed at: http://www.fda .gov/Drugs/GuidanceComplianceRegulatoryInformation/Surveillance /AdverseDrugEffects/ucm070434.htm.

4 **Incomplete reports in more than half of cases:** Institute for Safe Medical Practices. A critique of a key drug safety reporting system. January 28, 2015. Accessed at: http://www.ismp.org/quarterwatch/pdfs/2014Q1.pdf.

4 **Delay the reporting of many serious events:** Ma P, Marinovic I, Karaca-Mandic P. Drug manufacturers' delayed disclosure of serious and unexpected adverse events to the US Food and Drug Administration. *JAMA Intern Med.* 2015; 175: 1565–1566.

4 **The number of outpatient visits for adverse drug reactions:** Bourgeois FT, Shannon MW, Valim C, et al. Adverse drug events in the outpatient setting: an 11-Year national analysis. *Pharmacoepidemiol Drug Saf.* 2010; 19: 901–910.

6   **88,000 to 138,000 Americans had heart attacks from taking *Vioxx*:** US Senate (2004) Testimony of David J. Graham, MD. *MPH.* November 18, 2004. Washington, DC, USA: US Senate.

6   **The FDA fell so far behind in publishing these "watch lists":** Lowes R. Possible drug risks buried in delayed FDA "Watch Lists." *Medscape Medical News.* March 29, 2016. Accessed at: http://www.medscape.com /viewarticle/861078?nlid=102964_2863&src=wnl_dne_160330_-msc pedit&uac=26118EV&impID=1043236&faf=1#vp_1

7   **Increased risk of declining mental function:** Fox C, Richardson K, Maidment ID, et al. Anticholinergic medication use and cognitive impairment in the older population: the medical research council cognitive function and ageing study. *J Am Geriatr Soc.* 2011; 59: 1477–1483.

7   **Ten-year study of more than 3,000 people aged sixty-five and older:** Gray SL, Anderson ML, Dublin S, et al. Cumulative use of strong anticholinergics and incident dementia. *JAMA Intern Med.* 2015; 175: 401–407.

7   **Increased shrinking (atrophy) of several areas of the brain:** Risacher SL, McDonald BC, Tallman EF, et al. Association between anticholinergic medication use and cognition, brain metabolism, and brain atrophy in cognitively normal older adults. *JAMA Neurol.* Published online April 18, 2016. doi:10.1001/jamaneurol.2016.0580.

7   **Taking only one anticholinergic drug for just two months:** Cai X, Campbell N, Khan B, et al. Long-term anticholinergic use and the aging brain. *Alzheimer's & Dementia.* 2013; 9: 377–385.

8   **23,000 visits to emergency departments (EDs) and 2,000 hospitalizations:** Geller AL, Shehab N, Weidle NJ, et al. Emergency department visits for adverse events related to dietary supplements. *N Engl J Med.* 2015; 373: 1531–1540.

8.   **The use of five or more drugs nearly doubled:** Trends in prescription drug use among adults in the United States from 1999–2012. *JAMA.* 2015; 314: 1818–1830.

Drug-Drug Interactions

11   **If you take two different medications each day:** Delafuente JC. Understanding and preventing drug interactions in elderly patients. *Crit Rev Oncol Hematol.* 2003; 48: 133–143.

11 **Approximately 15.1 percent of older adults sixty-two to eighty-five:** Qato DM, Wilder J, Schumm LP, et al. Changes in prescription and over-the-counter medication and dietary supplement use among older adults in the United States, 2005 vs 2011. *JAMA Intern Med.* Published online March 21, 2016. doi:10.1001/jamainternmed.2015.8581.

12 **Warfarin along with the diabetes drugs:** Romley JA, Gong C, Jena AB, et al. Association between use of warfarin with common sulfonylureas and serious hypoglycemic events: retrospective cohort analysis. *BMJ.* 2015; 351: h6223.

12 **More than 7,000 people . . . 85 percent of physicians:** Boyer EW, Shannon M. The serotonin syndrome. *N Engl J Med.* 2005; 352: 1112–1120.

13 **Ginkgo biloba . . . St. John's wort:** Chen XW, Serag ES, Sneed KB, et al. Clinical herbal interactions with conventional drugs: from molecules to maladies. *Curr Med Chem.* 2011; 18 (31): 4836–4850.

Medication Errors

16 **7,000 Americans died:** Kohn K, Corrigan JM, Donaldson MS. *To Err is Human: Building a Safer Health System.* Washington, DC: National Academy of Sciences, National Academy Press; 2000.

16 **1.5 million people are harmed each year:** National Academies Institute of Medicine. Medication Errors Injure 1.5 Million People and Cost Billions of Dollars Annually. July 20, 2006. Accessed at: http://www8.nationalacademies.org/onpinews/newsitem.aspx?recordid=11623.

17 **The medical community does not want to publicly acknowledge:** Crowley CF, Nalder E. Within health care hides massive, avoidable death toll. *Hearst Newspapers.* August 9, 2009. Accessed at: http://www.seattlepi.com/national/article/Dead-by-Mistake-Within-health-care-hides-1305620.php.

17 **Average number of prescriptions written for people over age sixty-five nearly doubled:** Munson JC, Morden NE, Goodman DC, et al. *The Dartmouth Atlas of Medicare Prescription Drug Use.* Robert Wood Johnson Foundation. October, 2013. Accessed at: http://www.rwjf.org/en/library/research/2013/10/the-dartmouth-atlas-of-medicare-prescription-drug-use.html.

17 **Most common drugs that cause medical errors:** Wittich CM, Burkle CM, Lanier WL. Medication errors: an overview for clinicians. *Mayo Clin Proc.* 2014; 89: 1116–1125.

17 **Data analyzed from poison control centers:** Smith MD, Spiller HA, Casavant MJ, et al. Out-of-hospital medication errors among young children in the United States, 2002–2012. *Pediatrics.* 2014; 134: 867–876.

18 **Average of 66 minutes a day responding to electronic health records:** Murphy DR, Meyer AND, Russo E, et al. The burden of inbox notifications in commercial electronic health records. *JAMA Intern Med.* Published online March 14, 2016.

19 **34 percent of all prescriptions written in the United States:** American Public Health Association. Fact sheet: prescription medication use by older adults. Accessed at: www.medscape.com/viewarticle/501879.

20 **Study of nearly 500 adults ages fifty-five to seventy-four:** Wolf MS, Curtis LM, MS; Waite K, et al. Helping patients simplify and safely use complex prescription regimens. *Arch Intern Med.* 2011; 171: 300–305.

20 **Drug error rates of up to 42 percent:** Zimmerman S, Lover K, Sloane PD, et al. Medication administration errors in assisted living: scope, characteristics, and the importance of staff training. *J Am Geriatr Soc.* 2011; 59: 1060–1068.

21 **34 percent of all prescriptions written in the United States:** American Public Health Association. Fact sheet: prescription medication use by older adults. Accessed at: www.medscape.com/viewarticle/501879

21 **Misuse of NSAIDs:** Grissinger M. Top 10 adverse drug reactions and medication errors. Program and abstracts of the American Pharmacists Association 2007 Annual Meeting, March 16–19, Atlanta, Georgia; 2007.

21 **Accounts for more than 40 percent of acute liver failure cases in the United States:** Fontana RJ. Acute liver failure including acetaminophen overdose. *Med Clin North Am.* 2008; 92: 761–794.

21 **Drug overdoses surpassed traffic fatalities:** Warner M, Chen LH, Makuc DM, et al. Drug poisoning deaths in the United States, 1980–2008. *National Center for Health Statistics.* Data Brief No. 81, December 2011.

21 **By 2014, fatal overdoses reached 47,000:** Rudd RA, Aleshire N, JD; Zibbell JE, et al. Increases in drug and opioid overdose deaths—United States, 2000–2014. *CDC Morbidity and Mortality Weekly Report.* 2016; 64 (50); 1378–1382.

21 **In 2016, more than 64,000 Americans:** National Institute of Drug Abuse. Overdose death rates. Accessed at: https://www.drugabuse.gov/related-topics/trends-statistics/overdose-death-rates.

22 **CDC has recently released a strong warning to doctors:** FDA Drug Safety Communication: FDA warns about serious risks and death when combining opioid pain or cough medicines with benzodiazepines; requires its strongest warning. August 31, 2016. Accessed at: http://www.fda.gov/Drugs/DrugSafety/ucm518473.htm.

22 **Eighteen percent of twelfth graders:** National Institute of Drug Abuse. How many teens abuse prescription drugs? April 14, 2017. Accessed at: http://teens.drugabuse.gov/drug-facts/prescription-drugs.

Unnecessary and Inappropriate Drugs and Dosages

24 **The United States spends $200 billion each year:** Appleby J. Improper use of prescription drugs costs $200 billion a year, report finds. *Medscape Medical News.* June 20, 2013. Accessed at: http://www.medscape.com/viewarticle/806673.

24 **Nearly 60 percent of people over age sixty-five take at least one unnecessary drug:** Maher RL, Hanlon J, Hajjar ER. Clinical consequences of polypharmacy in elderly. *Expert Opin Drug Saf.* 2014; 13: 57–65.

26 **The most recent version published in 2015:** American Geriatrics Society. American Geriatrics Society 2015 updated Beers criteria for potentially inappropriate medication use in older adults. *J Am Geriatr Soc.* 2015; 63: 2227–2246.

26 **Increase the incidence of Alzheimer's disease by as much as 50 percent:** Billioti de Gage S, Moride Y, Decruet T, et al. Benzodiazepine use and risk of Alzheimer's disease: case-control study. *BMJ.* 2014; 349: g5205.

28 **Twenty-three million unnecessary antibiotic prescriptions:** Gonzales R, Steiner JF, Sande MA. Antibiotic prescribing for adults with colds, upper respiratory tract infections, and bronchitis by ambulatory care physicians. *JAMA.* 1997; 278: 901–904.

28 **Studies have shown that they work no better than sugar pills:** Fournier JC, DeRubeis RJ, Hollon SD, et al. Antidepressant drug effects and depression severity: a patient-level meta-analysis. *JAMA.* 2010; 303: 47–53.

29 **Up to 25 percent of middle-aged women:** Zhong W, Maradit-Kremers H, St. Sauver JL, et al. Age and sex patterns of drug prescribing in a defined American population. *Mayo Clin Proc.* 2013; 88: 697–707.

29 **The FDA recently issued a warning about an increased risk of hip, wrist, and spine fractures:** US Food and Drug Administration.

FDA Drug Safety Communication: Possible increased risk of fractures of the hip, wrist, and spine with the use of proton pump inhibitors. May 25, 2010. Accessed at: http://www.fda.gov/Drugs/DrugSafety /PostmarketDrugSafetyInformationforPatientsandProviders/ucm213206 .htm#SafetyAnnouncement.

29 **Audit of Medicare claims:** US Department of Health and Human Services. Medicare atypical antipsychotic drug claims for elderly nursing home residents. May 4, 2011. Accessed at: http://oig.hhs.gov/oei/reports /oei-07-08-00150.asp.

31 **In the book *Overdose:*** Cohen JS. *Overdose: the case against the drug companies.* New York: Jeremy P. Tarcher/Putnam; 2001.

33 ***Crestor,* which did not yet have a generic:** Brown T. Top 10 most prescribed generic drugs through September. *Medscape Medical News.* November 6, 2014. Accessed at: http://www.medscape.com/viewarticle/834578.

34 **Although there were fewer deaths from heart disease:** LaRosa, JC, Grundy, SM, Waters, DD, et al. Intensive lipid lowering with atorvastatin in patients with stable coronary disease. *N Engl J Med.* 2005; 352: 1425–1435.

34 **The FDA issued a safety alert:** US Food and Drug Administration. FDA Drug Safety Communication: New restrictions, contraindications, and dose limitations for Zocor (simvastatin) to reduce the risk of muscle injury. June 8, 2011. Accessed at: http://www.fda.gov/Drugs/DrugSafety /ucm256581.htm.

34 **Higher dose statin drugs have been found to be no better:** O'Brien EC, Wu J, Schulte PJ, et al. Statin use, intensity, and 3-year clinical outcomes among older patients with coronary artery disease. *Am Heart J.* 2016; 173: 27–34.

34 **Carrying an increased risk of side effects:** Silva M, Matthews ML, Jarvis C, et al. Meta-analysis of drug-induced adverse events associated with intensive-dose statin therapy. *Clin Ther.* 2007; 29: 253–260.

Chapter 2: Why We Are Taking So Many Pills
The Role of Big Pharma

36 **Accounting for nearly 17 percent of total health-care spending:** U.S. Department of Health and Human Services. Observations on trends in prescription drug spending. March 8, 2016. Accessed at: https://aspe.hhs .gov/pdf-report/observations-trends-prescription-drug-spending.

36 **This amounted to $1112:** Olson P, Sheiner L. The Hutchins Center explains: prescription drug spending. April 26, 2017. Accessed at: https://www.brookings.edu/blog/up-front/2017/04/26/the-hutchins-center-explains-prescription-drug-spending/.

37 **$14 million a day:** Healthcare marketing. Advertising Age. October 17, 2016. Accessed at: http://gaia.adage.com/images/bin/pdf/KantarHCwhitepaper_complete.pdf.

37 **The average American TV viewer sees nine drug advertisements:** Ventola CL. Direct-to-Consumer pharmaceutical advertising: therapeutic or toxic? *Pharm Ther*. 2011; 36: 669–674, 681–684.

38 **Requests were made during about 40 percent of doctor visits:** Lee AL. Who are the opinion leaders? The physicians, pharmacists, patients and direct-to-consumer advertising. *J Health Commun*. 2010; 15: 629–655.

38 **Ten percent of men cannot achieve a full erection:** Connors AL. Big bad pharma: An ethical analysis of physician-directed and consumer-directed marketing tactics. *Albany Law Rev*. 2009; 73: 243–282.

38 **Member of an FDA advisory panel told a reporter about a heavily advertised new sleep medication:** Cohn J. Drugs you don't need for disorders you don't have. *The Huffington Post*. March 2016. Accessed at: http://highline.huffingtonpost.com/articles/en/sleep-advertising/.

39 **The FDA received more than 1,000 complaints:** Institute for Safe Medical Practices. Monitoring FDA MedWatch reports. January 13, 2016. Accessed at: https://www.ismp.org/quarterwatch/pdfs/2015Q2.pdf.

40 **Research evidence for this new drug, Ditropan:** Agency for Healthcare Quality and Research. Treatment of overactive bladder in women. *Evidence Report/Technology Assessment Number 187*. 2009. Accessed at: http://www.ahrq.gov/downloads/pub/evidence/pdf/bladder/bladder.pdf.

40 **Shannon Brownlee, in her excellent book:** Brownlee S. *Overtreated: Why Too Much Medicine Is Making Us Sicker and Poorer*. New York: Bloomsbury USA; 2007.

43 **The FDA cites inadequate staffing and competing priorities:** Lowes R. Possible drug risks buried in delayed FDA "Watch Lists." *Medscape Medical News*. March 29, 2016. Accessed at: http://www.medscape.com/viewarticle/861078?

43 **An investigative journalism team from New York University:** Seife C. Are your medications safe? The FDA buries evidence of fraud in

medical trials. February 9, 2015. Available at: http://www.slate.com/articles /health_and_science/science/2015/02/fda_inspections_fraud_fabrication _and_scientific_misconduct_are_hidden_from.html.

43   **More than 60 percent of its funding from the pharmaceutical industry**: Tavernise S. FDA nominee Califf's ties to drug makers worry some. *New York Times.* September 19, 2015. Accessed at: http://www.nytimes .com/2015/09/20/health/fda-nominee-califfs-ties-to-drug-industry-raise -questions.html?_r=1.

43   **Relationships have led many public health advocates:** Public Citizen. Senate should reject President's nominee to be the next FDA commissioner. Published September 16, 2015. Accessed at: http://www.citizen .org/pressroom/pressroomredirect.cfm?ID=5635.

43   **The industry spent nearly $150 million lobbying Congress:** Center for Responsive Politics. Pharmaceutical manufacturing industry profile: summary, 2015. Accessed at: http://www.opensecrets.org/lobby/induscode .php?id=H4300&year=2015.

44   **Money paid to doctors from drug companies:** Ornstein C, Groeger L, Tigas M, et al. Dollars for docs. December 13, 2016. Accessed at: https: //projects.propublica.org/docdollars/.

45   **Pfizer . . . paid nearly $128 million to 168,928 doctors:** as above. Accessed at https://projects.propublica.org/docdollars/company/pfizer-inc.

45   **Story of a first-year Harvard medical student:** Wilson D. Harvard medical school in ethics quandary. *New York Times.* March 2, 2009. Accessed at: http://www.nytimes.com/2009/03/03/business/03medschool.html?hp.

45   **Nine-member panel that included six who had received research grants:** Kassirer JP. Why should we swallow what these studies say? *Washington Post.* August 1, 2004. Accessed at: http://www.washingtonpost .com/wp-dyn/articles/A29456-2004Jul31.html.

45   **Panels making recommendations for treatment of high blood pressure and obesity:** Wilson D. Health Guideline Panels Struggle with Conflicts of Interest. *New York Times.* November 2, 2011. Accessed at: http://www .nytimes.com/2011/11/03/health/policy/health-guideline-panels -struggle-with-conflicts-of-interest.html?_r=0.

46   **$24 billion spent on direct physician marketing:** Pew Charitable Trusts. Persuading the prescribers: pharmaceutical industry marketing and its influence on physicians and patients. November 11, 2013. Accessed at: http://

www.pewtrusts.org/en/research-and-analysis/fact-sheets/2013/11/11/
persuading-the-prescribers-pharmaceutical-industry-market
ing-and-its-influence-on-physicians-and-patients.

46 **Association between payments or gifts physicians receive:** Yeh JS,
Franklin JM, Avorn J, et al. Association of industry payments to physicians
with the prescribing of brand-name statins in Massachusetts. *JAMA Intern
Med.* 2016; 176: 763–768.

46 **According to Open Payments:** Types and distribution of payments from
industry to physicians in 2015. *JAMA.* 2017; 31: 1774–1778.

47 **Faculty members at many top medical institutions who can net
tens of thousands of dollars:** Weber T, Ornstein C. Med schools flunk
at keeping faculty off Pharma speaking circuit. *Pro Publica.* December 19,
2010. Available at: https://www.propublica.org/article/medical-schools
-policies-on-faculty-and-drug-company-speaking-circuit.

47 **Drug-company-funded studies that have positive results:** Bourgeois FT,
Murthy S, Mandl KD. Outcome reporting among drug trials registered in
Clinical Trials.gov. *Ann Intern Med.* 2010; 153: 158–166.

47 **Studies funded by pharmaceutical companies are also more likely to
show a benefit:** Ridker PM, Torres J. Reported outcomes in major cardiovascular clinical trials funded by for-profit and not-for-profit organizations: 2000–2005. *JAMA.* 2006; 295 (19): 2270–2274.

47 **Analysis of seventy-four FDA-registered studies of antidepressants:**
Turner EH, Matthews AM, Linardatos E, et al. Selective publication of
antidepressant trials and its influence on apparent efficacy. *NEJM.* 2008;
358: 252–260.

48 **A study of fifty-seven published trials:** Seife C. Research Misconduct
Identified by the US Food and Drug Administration. *JAMA Intern Med.*
2015; 175 (4): 567–577.

48 **Editor of the highly regarded medical journal** *The Lancet:* Horton R.
Comment Offline: What is medicines 5 sigma? *The Lancet.* 2015; 385:
1380.

49 **The recently-approved drug** *Addyi* **. . . is a case in point:** Thomas K, Mor-
genson G. The female Viagra, undone by a drug maker's dysfunction. *New
York Times.* April 9, 2016. Available at: http://www.nytimes.com/2016/04/10
/business/female-viagra-addyi-valeant-dysfunction.html?_r=0.

49 **Women taking the drug also had four times as much dizziness:** Jaspers L, Feys F, Bramer WM, et al. Efficacy and safety of flibanserin for the treatment of hypoactive sexual desire disorder in women: a systematic review and meta-analysis. *JAMA Intern Med.* 2016; 176 (4) :453–462.

49 **Study of 14,000 patients in forty-five countries:** Project on Government Oversight. Drug problems: Nominee to head FDA led clinical trial FDA faulted. November 12, 2015. Available at: http://www.pogo.org /blog/2015/11/fda-nominee-robert-califf-led-faulted-fda-trial.html.

49 **Commercial sponsors of these clinical trials may not be motivated:** Finegold JA, Manisly CH, Goldacre B, et al. What proportion of symptomatic side effects in patients taking statins are genuinely caused by the drug? *Eur J Prev Cardiol.* 2014; 21: 464–474.

50 **Study funded by the German government:** Wieseler B, Wolfram N, McGauran N, et al. Completeness of reporting of patient-relevant clinical trial outcomes: comparison of unpublished clinical study reports with publicly available data. *PLoS One.* 2013. https://doi.org/10.1371/journal .pmed.1001526.

50 **More than 95 percent of the advertising that keeps them afloat:** Washington HA. Flacking for Big Pharma. The American Scholar. June 3, 2011. Available at: https://theamericanscholar.org/flacking-for-big-pharma/#.Vwbc 4-YYHlo

The Role of Doctors

51 **A recent study of internal medicine residents:** Hill RG, Sears LM, -Melanson SW. 4000 clicks: a productivity analysis of electronic medical records in a community hospital ED. *Am J Emerg Med.* 2013; 31: 1591–1594.

51 **Physician burnout and creating problems with their personal relationships:** Dyrbye LN, Sotile W, Boone S, et al. A survey of U.S. physicians and their partners regarding the impact of work–home conflict. *J Gen Int Med.* 2014; 29: 155–161.

51 **Doctors counseled their patients about:** Ritsema TS, Bingenheimer JB, Scholting P, et al. Differences in the delivery of health education to patients with chronic disease by provider type, 2005–2009. *Prev Chronic Dis.* 2014; 11: 130175.

52 **Medicare saved $2,650 for each person:** Pear R. Medicare proposal takes aim at diabetes. *New York Times.* March 23, 2016. Accessed at: http://www .nytimes.com/2016/03/23/us/politics/medicare-proposal-takes-aim-at -diabetes.html?smprod=nytcore-iphone&smid=nytcore-iphone-share& _r=0.

Chapter 3: High Cholesterol and Cardiovascular Disease

59 **One out of every three deaths in the United States:** Mozaffarian D, Benjamin EJ, Go AS, et al. Heart disease and stroke statistics—2015 update: a report from the American Heart Association. *Circulation.* 2015; 131: e29-e322.

59 **Among brand-name drugs:** Brown T. The 10 most-prescribed and top-selling medications. *WebMD.* May 8, 2015. Accessed at: www.webmd .com/drug-medication/news/20150508/most-prescribed-top-selling-drugs.

60 **One-quarter of all Americans aged forty and above:** Gu Q, Paulose-Ram R, Burt VL, et al. Prescription cholestrol-lowering medication use in adults aged 40 and over: United States, 2003–2012. National Center for Health Statistics Data Brief No.177. December 2014. Accessed at: https://www .cdc.gov/nchs/data/databriefs/db177.pdf.

60 **More than half of all men and 40 percent of all women aged sixty-five and older:** Centers for Disease Control and Prevention. Health, United States, 2012. Table 92. Accessed at http://www.cdc.gov/nchs/data /hus/2012/092.pdf.

60 **Overall, an estimated 38.6 million Americans are taking a statin:** Adedinsewo D, Taka N, Agasthi P, et al. Prevalence and factors associated with statin use among a nationally representative sample of US adults: National Health and Nutrition Examination Survey, 2011–2012. *Clin Cardiol.* 2016: 39: 491–496.

60 **Nearly everyone over age fifty should take these cholesterol-lowering drugs:** Ebrahim S, Casas JP. Statins for all by the age of 50 years? *Lancet.* 2012; 380: 545–547.

61 **Study of diet and heart disease in seven countries:** Keys A (ed). Coronary heart disease in seven countries. *Circulation.* 1970: 41: s1–211.

61 **72 percent of them did not have high cholesterol:** Canto JG, Kiefe CI, Rogers WJ, et al. Number of coronary heart disease risk factors and

mortality in patients with first myocardial infarction. *JAMA*. 2011; 306: 2120–2127.

61 **An analysis of twenty-one studies involving nearly 350,000 people:** Siri-Tarino PW, Sun Q, Hu FB, et al. Meta-analysis of prospective cohort studies evaluating the association of saturated fat with cardiovascular disease. *Am J Clin Nutr*. 2010; 91: 535–546.

61 **The American Heart Association released an advisory:** Sacks FM, Lichtenstein AH, Wu JHY, et al. Dietary fats and cardiovascular disease: a presidential advisory from the American Heart Association. *Circulation*. 2017; CIRC.0000000000000510. Published online June 15, 2017.

61 **Association between a marker of inflammation in the blood:** Koenig W, Frohlich M, Fischer H-G, et al. C-Reactive Protein, a sensitive marker of inflammation, predicts future risk of coronary heart disease in initially healthy middle-aged men. *Circulation*. 1999; 99: 237–242.

62 **Report published in September 2016 revealed that the sugar industry:** Kearns CE, Schmidt LA, Glantz SA. Sugar industry and coronary heart disease research: A historical analysis of internal industry documents. *JAMA Intern Med*. 2016. doi: 10.1001/jamainternmed.2016.5394.

62 **Decreasing the saturated fat in our diets has actually increased the risk:** Malhotra A. Saturated fat is not the major issue: let's bust the myth of its role in heart disease. *BMJ*. 2013; 347: f6340.

63 **Eighty percent of cardiovascular disease could be prevented:** Yusuf S, Hawken S, Ounpuu S, et al. Effect of potentially modifiable risk factors associated with myocardial infarction in 52 countries (the INTERHEART study): case-control study. *Lancet*. 2004; 364: 937–952.

63 **Lifestyle modifications could reduce the risk of CVD in women:** Stampfer MJ, Hu FB, Manson JE, et al. Primary prevention of coronary heart disease in women through diet and lifestyle. *N Engl J Med*. 2000; 343: 16–22.

64 **Consuming a Mediterranean diet . . . can reduce heart disease and deaths:** Estruch R, Ros E, Salas-Salvado J, et al. Primary Prevention of Cardiovascular Disease with a Mediterranean Diet. *N Engl J Med*. 2013; 368: 1279–1290; and Samieri C, Sun Q, Townsend MK, et al. The association between dietary patterns at midlife and health in aging: an observational Study. *Ann Intern Med*. 2013; 159: 584–591.

64 **25 percent reduction that has been attributed to statin drugs:** Taylor F, Huffman MD, Macedo A, et al. Statins for the primary prevention of cardiovascular disease. *Cochrane Database Syst Rev.* 2013; 1: CD004816.

64 **The more fiber that is eaten:** Greenwood DC, Evans CEL, Cleghorn CL, et al. Dietary fibre intake and risk of cardiovascular disease: systematic review and meta-analysis. *BMJ.* 2013; 347: f6879.

64 **For every seven grams of fiber eaten each day:** Wu H, Flint AJ, Qi Q, et al. Association between dietary whole-grain intake and risk of mortality: two large prospective studies in US men and women. *JAMA Intern Med.* 2015; 175: 373–384.

64 **If everyone over age fifty in Great Britain ate only one apple a day:** Briggs ADM, Mizdrak A, Scarborough P, et al. A statin a day keeps the doctor away: comparative proverb assessment modelling study. *BMJ.* 2013; 347: f7267.

65 **Drinking as little as one extra soft drink each day:** Yang Q, Zhang Z, Gregg EW, et al. Added sugar intake and cardiovascular diseases mortality among US adults. *JAMA Intern Med.* 2014; 174: 516–524.

65 **Study of more than 75,000 healthy middle-aged women:** Liu S, Willett WC, Stampfer MJ, et al. A prospective study of dietary glycemic load, carbohydrate intake, and risk of coronary heart disease in US women. *Am J Clin Nutr.* 2000; 71: 1455–1461.

65 **Study of more than 117,000 Chinese men and women:** Yu D, Shu X-O, Li H, et al. Dietary carbohydrates, refined grains, glycemic load, and risk of coronary heart disease in Chinese adults. *Am J Epidemiol.* 2013; 178: 1542–1549.

65 **Those with low fitness had nearly twice the risk of death:** Wickramasinghe CD, Ayers CR, Das S. Prediction of 30-year risk for cardiovascular mortality by fitness and risk factor levels: the Cooper Center Longitudinal Study. *Circ Cardiovasc Qual Outcomes.* 2014; 7: 597–602.

66 **A 64 percent increased risk of dying:** Warren TY, Barry V, Hooker SP, et al. Sedentary behaviors increase risk of cardiovascular disease mortality in men. *Med Sci Sports Exerc.* 2010; 42: 8790885.

66 **Replacing sitting with light activities:** Beddhu S, Wei G, Marcus RL, et al. Light-intensity physical activities and mortality in the United States general population and CKD subpopulation. *Clin J Am Soc Nephrol.* 2015; 10: 1145–1153.

66 **Only one in three adults in the United States get the recommended amount**: President's Council on Fitness, Sports & Nutrition. Available at: http://www.fitness.gov/resource-center/facts-and-statistics/#footnote-3.

66 **Sixty-six percent of US women and 75 percent of men are overweight:** Yang L, Colditz GA. Prevalence of overweight and obesity in the United States, 2007–2012. *JAMA Intern Med.* 2015; 175: 1412–1413.

66 **People with a normal BMI but central obesity:** Coutinho T, Goel K, Correa de Sá D, et al. Combining body mass index with measures of central obesity in the assessment of mortality in subjects with coronary heart disease. Role of "normal weight central obesity." *J Am Coll Cardiol.* 2012; 61: 553–560.

67 **Statin users consumed about 200 calories more per day:** Sugiyama T, Tsugawa Y, Tseng CH, et al. Different time trends of caloric and fat intake between statin users and nonusers among US adults. *JAMA Intern Med.* 2014; 174: 1038–1045.

67 **Long-term smokers aged sixty and over who quit smoking:** Mons U, Müezzinler A, Gellert C, et al. Impact of smoking and smoking cessation on cardiovascular events and mortality in older adults: meta-analysis of individual participant data from prospective cohort studies of the CHANCES consortium. *BMJ.* 2015; 350: h1551.

67 **High stress was found to be associated with a 27 percent increase in coronary heart disease:** Richardson S, Shaffer JA, Falzon L, et al. Meta-analysis of perceived stress and its association with incident coronary heart disease. *Am J Cardiol.* 2012; 110: 1711–1716.

67 **The risk of heart attacks increased nearly fivefold:** Mostofsky E, Penner EA, Mittleman MA, et al. Outbursts of anger as a trigger of acute cardiovascular events: a systematic review and meta-analysis. *Eur Heart J.* 2014; 35: 1404–1410.

68 **Using drugs to treat depression:** Zuidersma M, Conradi HJ, van Melle JP, et al. Depression treatment after myocardial infarction and long-term risk of subsequent cardiovascular events and mortality: a randomized controlled trial. *J Psychosom Res.* 2013; 74: 25–30.

68 **Study of 237 Swedish women with coronary heart disease:** Orth-Gomer K, Schneiderman N, Wang HX, et al. Stress reduction prolongs life in women with coronary disease: the Stockholm Women's Intervention Trial for Coronary Heart Disease (SWITCHD). *Circ Cardiovasc Qual Outcomes.* 2009; 2: 25–32.

69 **Various natural interventions have been shown to lower LDL cholesterol:** Sorrentino MJ. An update on statin alternatives and adjuncts. *Clin Lipidology.* 2012; 7:721–730.

69 **Apple cider vinegar lowered cholesterol levels:** Shishehbor F, Mansoori A, Sarkaki AR, et al. Apple cider vinegar attenuates lipid profile in normal and diabetic rats. *Pak J Biol Sci.* 2008; 11: 2634–2638.

69 **High doses of niacin, also known as vitamin B_3, lowered LDL cholesterol:** Boden WE, Sidhu MS, Toth PP. The therapeutic role of niacin in dyslipidemia management. *J Cardiovasc Pharmacol Ther.* 2014; 19: 141–158.

69 **Red yeast rice, a traditional Chinese medicine:** Venero CV, Venero JV, Wortham DC, et al. Lipid-lowering efficacy of red yeast rice in a population intolerant to statins. *Am J Cardiol.* 2010; 105: 664–666.

69 **Survey of twelve commercially available red yeast rice products:** Gordon RY, Cooperman T, Obermeyer W, et al. Marked variability of monacolin levels in commercial red yeast rice products: buyer beware! *Arch Intern Med.* 2010; 170: 1722–1727.

70 **A head-to-head study of rosuvastatin:** Nicholls SJ, Ballantyne CM, Barter PJ, et al. Effect of two intensive statin regimens on progression of coronary disease. *N Engl J Med.* 2011; 365: 2078–2087.

71 **A randomized trial of nearly 2,900 adults aged sixty-five:** Han BH, Sutin D, Williamson JD, et al. Effect of statin treatment vs usual care on primary cardiovascular prevention among older adults. *JAMA Intern Med.* doi:10.1001/jamainternmed.2017.1442.

71 **For every eighty-three people treated for five years with a statin:** Newman D. Statins given for 5 years for heart disease prevention (with known heart disease). *The NNT.* July 17, 2015. Accessed at: http://www.thennt .com/nnt/statins-for-heart-disease-prevention-with-known-heart-disease/.

71 **140 of these people would have to be treated with statins for five years:** Abramson JD, Rosenberg HG, Jewell N, et al. Should people at low risk of cardiovascular disease take a statin? *BMJ.* 2013; 347: f6123.

72 **Of the nine members of the panel that wrote the guidelines:** Kassirer JP. Why should we swallow what these studies say? *Washington Post.* August 1, 2004. Accessed at: http://www.washingtonpost.com/wp-dyn/articles /A29456-2004Jul31.html.

72 **LDL cholesterol should be the major factor:** Raymond C, Cho L, Rocco M, et al. New cholesterol guidelines: worth the wait? *Cleve Clin J Med.* 2014; 81: 11–19.

73 **The calculator overestimated the risk of cardiovascular events:** DeFilippis AP, Young R, Carrubba CJ, et al. An analysis of calibration and discrimination among multiple cardiovascular risk scores in a modern multiethnic cohort. *Ann Intern Med.* 2015; 162: 266–275.

74 **Almost one in five patients stop taking statins:** Zhang H, Plutzky J, Skentzos S, et al. Discontinuation of statins in routine care settings. *Ann Intern Med.* 2013; 158: 526–534.

74 **7 to 29 percent of statin users had muscle symptoms:** Stroes ES, Thompson PD, Corsini A, et al. Statin-associated muscle symptoms: impact on statin therapy. European Atherosclerosis Society Consensus Panel Statement on Assessment, Aetiology and Management. *Eur Heart J.* 2015; 36: 1012–1022.

74 **More likely to have injuries such as sprains, strains, and dislocations:** Mansi I, Frei CR, Pugh MJ, et al. Statins and musculoskeletal conditions, arthropathies, and injuries. *JAMA Intern Med.* 2013; 173: 1318–1326.

74 **Twice as much muscle damage after running on a treadmill:** Bouitbir J, Charles AL, Rasseneur L, et al. Atorvastatin treatment reduces exercise capacities in rats: involvement of mitochondrial impairments and oxidative stress. *J Appl Physiol (1985).* 2011; 111: 1477–1483.

74 **Statins also can impair the functioning of the heart muscle itself:** Rubinstein J, Aloka F, Abela GS. Statin therapy decreases myocardial function as evaluated via strain imaging. *Clin Cardiol.* 2009; 32: 684–689.

74 **Taking statins along with other medications:** Ito MK, Maki KC, Brinton EA, et al. Muscle symptoms in statin users, associations with cytochrome P450, and membrane transporter inhibitor use: a subanalysis of the USAGE study. *J Clin Lipidol.* 2014; 8: 69–76.

76 **In 2012, the FDA issued a safety announcement:** US Food and Drug Administration. FDA Drug Safety Communication: Important safety label changes to cholesterol-lowering statin drugs. February 28, 2012. Accessed at: http://www.fda.gov/Drugs/DrugSafety/ucm293101.htm.

76 **Survey of statin patients who experienced cognitive problems:** Evans MA, Golomb BA. Statin-associated adverse cognitive effects: survey results from 171 patients. *Pharmacotherapy.* 2009; 29: 800–811.

76   **Compelling evidence about the effect of statins on memory loss:** Strom BL, Schinnar R, Karlawish J, et al. Statin therapy and risk of acute memory impairment. *JAMA Intern Med.* 2015; 175: 1399–1405.

76   **A study of people aged seventy and above:** Mielke MM, Zandi PP, Sjogren M, et al. High total cholesterol levels in late life associated with a reduced risk of dementia. *Neurology.* 2005; 64: 1689–1695.

77   **Alzheimers Association estimates that one in ten people aged sixty-five and over:** http://www.alz.org/facts/overview.asp.

78   **Women on all types of statin drugs:** Culver AL, Ockene IS, Balasubramanian R, et al. Statin use and risk of diabetes mellitus in postmenopausal women in the Women's Health Initiative. *Arch Intern Med.* 2012; 172: 144–152.

78   **Followed more than 8,700 nondiabetic patients for nearly six years:** Cederberg H, Stancakova A, Yaluri N, et al. Increased risk of diabetes with statin treatment is associated with impaired insulin sensitivity and insulin secretion: a six-year follow-up study of the METSIM cohort. *Diabetologia.* 2015; 58: 1109–1117.

78   **Nearly a twofold increase in developing new onset diabetes:** Mansi I, Frei CR, Wang C-P, et al. Statins and new-onset diabetes mellitus and diabetic complications: a retrospective cohort study of US healthy adults. *J Gen Intern Med.* 2015; 30: 1599–1610.

78   **Data from a large military health-care system:** Leuschen J, Mortensen EM, Frei CR, et al. Association of statin use with cataracts: a propensity score-matched analysis. *JAMA Ophthalmol.* 2013; 131: 1427–1434.

78   **Canadian study found a 48 percent increased risk of cataracts:** Machan CM, Hrynchak PK, Irving EL. Age-related cataract is associated with type diabetes and statin use. *Optom Vis Sci.* 2012; 89: 1165–1171.

79   **Macular degeneration, another age-related eye disease:** VanderBeek BL, Zacks DN, Talwar N, et al. Role of statins in the development and progression of age-related macular degeneration. *Retina.* 2013; 33: 414–422.

79   **Statins users have on average one-and-a-half times the risk of moderate or severe liver damage:** Hippisley-Cox J, Coupland C. Unintended effects of statins in men and women in England and Wales: population based cohort study using the QResearch database. *BMJ.* 2010; 340: c2197.

79   **Researchers estimate that excessive fatigue affects between 20 and 40 percent:** Golomb BA, Evans MA, Dimsdale JE, et al. Effects of statins on

energy and fatigue with exertion: results from a randomized controlled trial. *Arch Intern Med.* 2012; 172: 1180–1182.

79 **Mood disorders and even suicide:** De Berardis D, Conti CM, Serroni N, et al. The role of cholesterol levels in mood disorders and suicide. *J Biol Regul Homeost Agents.* 2009; 23: 133–140.

79 **30 percent increased risk back disorders:** Makris UE, Alvarz CA, Wei W, et al. Association of statin use with risk of back disorder diagnoses. Research Letter. *JAMA Intern Med.* 2017; doi:10.1001/jamainternmed.2017.1068.

79 **There is preliminary evidence of other side effects associated with statins:** Golumb BA, Evans BS. Statin adverse effects: a review of the literature and evidence for a mitochondrial mechanism. *Am J Cardiovasc Drugs.* 2008; 8: 373–418.

81 **Supplementation with coenzyme Q10 can alleviate the muscle pains:** Littlefield N, Beckstrand RL, Luthy KE. Statins' effect on plasma levels of Coenzyme Q10 and improvement in myopathy with supplementation. *J Am Assoc Nurse Pract.* 2014; 26:85–90.

Chapter 4: Osteoporosis

82 **Seventy percent of people over age eighty:** World Health Federation. Chronic rheumatic conditions: osteoporosis. Accessed at: http://www.who .int/chp/topics/rheumatic/en/.

82 **Estimated to reach $9 billion by 2020:** Transparency Market Research. Osteoporosis drugs market to grow at 1.2 percent CAGR by 2020, driven by rising occurrence of osteoporosis. September 14, 2015. Accessed at http://www.transparencymarketresearch.com/pressrelease/osteoporosis -drugs-market.htm.

83 **Financial support from several pharmaceutical companies:** Alonso-Coello P, Garcia-Franco AL, Guyatt G, et al. Drugs for pre-osteoporosis: prevention or disease mongering? *BMJ.* 2008; 336: 126–129.

83 **Almost 44 percent of US adults aged fifty years and older:** Wright NC, Looker AC, Saag KG, et al. The recent prevalence of osteoporosis and low bone mass in the United States based on bone mineral density at the femoral neck or lumbar spine. *J Bone Miner Res.* 2014; 29: 2520–2526.

84 **Using the FRAX calculator, it is recommended that almost three-fourths:** Donaldson MG, Cawthon PM, Lui LY, et al. Estimates of the proportion of older white women who would be recommended for

pharmacologic treatment by the new US National Osteoporosis Foundation Guidelines. *J Bone Miner Res.* 2009; 24: 675–680.

84 **According to the American Board of Internal Medicine:** Choosing Wisely. Bone-Density Tests: when you need a test and when you don't. May, 2012. Accessed at: http://www.choosingwisely.org/patient-resources /bone-density-tests/.

84 **Twenty to thirty percent of people with hip fractures die within one year:** Castronuovo E. Pezzotti P, Franzo A, et al. Early and late mortality in elederly patients after hip fracture: a cohort study using administrative health databases in the Lazio region, Italy. *BMC Geriatr.* 2011; 11: 37. doi:10.1186/1471-2318-11-37.

84 **Published in the top-ranking *British Medical Journal:*** Järvinen TLN, Michaëlsson K, Jokihaara J, et al. Overdiagnosis of bone fragility in the quest to prevent hip fracture. *BMJ.* 2015; 350: h2088.

86 **The recommended amount of calcium:** Institute of Medicine. DRIs for calcium and vitamin D. November 30, 2010, Accessed at: http://iom .nationalacademies.org/Reports/2010/Dietary-Reference-Intakes-for -Calcium-and-Vitamin-D/DRI-Values.aspx.

86 **Experts at an international meeting about osteoporosis:** Harvey NC, Biver E, *Kaufman* JM, et al. The role of calcium supplementation in healthy musculoskeletal ageing: an expert consensus meeting of the European Society for Clinical and Economic Aspects of Osteoporosis, Osteoarthritis, and Musculoskeletal Diseases (ESCEO) and the International Foundation for Osteoporosis (IOF). *Osteoporos Int.* 2017; 28: 447–462.

88 **Avoiding the sun was as much of a risk factor:** Lindqvist PG, Epstein E, Nielsen K, et al. Avoidance of sun exposure as a risk factor for major causes of death: a competing risk analysis of the Melanoma in Southern Sweden cohort. *J Int Med.* 2016 Mar 16. doi:10.1111/joim.12496.

88 **Data from ninety-five different studies:** Chowdhury R, Kunutsor S, Vitezova A, et al. Vitamin D and risk of cause specific death: systematic review and meta-analysis of observational cohort and randomised intervention studies. *BMJ.* 2014; 348: g1903.

88 **Elderly patients with vitamin D deficiency:** Miller JW, Harvey DJ, Beckett LA, et al. Vitamin D status and rates of cognitive decline in a multiethnic cohort of older adults. *JAMA Neurol.* 2015; 72: 1295–1303.

88 **Age-related macular degeneration (AMD):** Annweiler C, Drouet M, Duva GT, et al. Circulating vitamin D concentration and age-related macular degeneration: systematic review and meta-analysis. *Maturitis.* 2016; 88: 101–112.

88 **A blood serum level of 40 to 50 nanograms/milliliter:** Baggerly CA, Cuomo RE, French CB, et al. Sunlight and vitamin D: necessary for public health. *J Am Coll of Nutr.* 2015; 34: 359–365.

89 **Endocrine Society recommends:** Holick MF, Binkley NC, Bischoff-Ferrari HA, et al. Evaluation, treatment, and prevention of vitamin D deficiency: an Endocrine Society Clinical Practice guideline. *J Clin Endocrin Metab.* 2011; 96: 1911–1930.

90 **Smoking decreases bone mass:** Wong PK, Chrisstie JJ, Wark JD. The effects of smoking on bone health. *Clin Sci (Lond).* 2007; 113: 233–241.

90 **More than two drinks per day:** Berg KM, -Kunins HV, Jackson JL, et al. Association between alcohol consumption and both osteoporotic fracture and bone density. *Am J Med.* 2008; 121: 406–418.

90 **Large amounts of caffeine:** Rapuri PB, Gallagher JC, Kinyamu HK. Caffeine intake increases the rate of bone loss in elderly women and interacts with vitamin D receptor genotypes. *Amer J Clin Nutr.* 2001; 74: 694–700.

90 **Study published in 2006 found that:** Tucker KL, Morita K, Qiao N, et al. Colas, but not other carbonated beverages, are associated with low bone mineral density in older women: The Framingham Osteoporosis Study. *Am J Clin Nutr.* 2006; 84: 936–942.

90 **A thirty-year study of nearly 75,000 postmenopausal women:** Fung TT, Arasaratman MH, Grodstein F, et al. Soda consumption and risk of hip fractures in postmenopausal women in the Nurses' Health Study. *Am J Clin Nutr.* 2014; 100: 953–958.

90 **Steroid drugs such as prednisone:** Canalis E, Mazziotti G, Giustina A, et al. Glucocorticoid-induced osteoporosis: pathophysiology and therapy. *Osteoporos Int.* 2007; 18: 1319–1328.

91 **Correlation between steroids, used by 2.5 percent:** van Staa TP, Leufkens HG, Abenhaim L, et al. Use of oral corticosteroids and risk of fractures. *J Bone Miner Res.* 2000; 15: 993–1000.

91 **Older women taking PPIs have an increased risk:** *Cai D, Feng W, Jiang Q.* Acid-suppressive medications and risk of fracture: an updated meta-analysis. *Int J Clin Exp Med.* 2015; 8: 8893–8904.

91 **Selective serotonin reuptake inhibitor (SSRI) antidepressants:** Rizzoli R, Cooper C, Reginster JY, et al. Antidepressant medications and osteoporosis. *Bone.* 2012; 51: 606–613.

91 **SSRIs were found to cause an even higher risk:** Melville NA. SSRI Fracture Risk Exceeds That of Corticosteroids and PPIs. *Medscape Medical News.* October 7, 2013. Accessed at: http://www.medscape.com/viewarticle /812176.

91 **Thiazolidinedione diabetes drugs:** Raz I. Guideline approach to therapy in patients with newly diagnosed type 2 diabetes. *Diabetes Care.* 2013; 36: Supplement 2.

91 **Antiepileptic drugs:** Petty SJ, O'Brien TJ, Wark JD. Antiepileptic medication and bone health. *Osteopor Int.* 2007; 18: 129–142.

91 **Anti-coagulants like warfarin:** Gage BF, Birman-Deych E, Radford MJ, et al. Risk of osteoporotic fracture in elderly patients taking warfarin. *Arch Intern Med.* 2006; 166: 241–246.

91 **Half of the twenty most commonly prescribed medications:** Kuschel BM, Laflamme L, Möller J. The risk of fall injury in relation to commonly prescribed medications among older people—a Swedish case-control study. *Eur J Pub Health.* 2015; 25: 527–532.

92 **A Canadian study found no difference:** Crilly RG, Kloseck M, Chesworth B. Comparison of hip fracture and osteoporosis medication prescription rates across Canadian provinces. *Osteoporos Int.* 2014; 25: 205–210.

93 **Another study of the risk of hip fractures in women aged sixty-five and over:** Erviti J, Alonso A, Gorricho J, et al. Oral bisphosphonates may not decrease hip fracture risk in elderly Spanish women: a nested case–control study. *BMJ Open.* 2013; 3: e002084.

93 **FDA cautions doctors:** US Food and Drug Administration. Information for Healthcare Professionals: Bisphosphonates (marketed as Actonel, Actonel+Ca, Aredia, Boniva, Didronel, Fosamax, Fosamax+D, Reclast, Skelid, and Zometa). August 15, 2013. Accessed at: http://www.fda.gov /Drugs/DrugSafety/PostmarketDrugSafetyInformationforPatientsand Providers/ucm124165.htm.

93 **Up to 20 percent of people stop taking bisphosphonates:** Reid IR. Bisphosphonates in the treatment of osteoporosis: a review of their contribution and controversies. *Skelet Radiol.* 2011; 40: 1191–1196.

93 **FDA issued a safety announcement:** US Food and Drug Administration. FDA Drug Safety Communication: Safety update for osteoporosis drugs, bisphosphonates, and atypical fractures. October 13, 2010. Accessed at: http://www.fda.gov/Drugs/DrugSafety/ucm229009.htm.

94 **Microscopic cracks that develop from suppressing:** Saita Y, Ishijima M, Kaneko K. Atypical femoral fractures and bisphosphonate use: current evidence and clinical implications. *Ther Adv Chronic Dis.* 2015; 6: 185–193.

94 **The longer one takes these medications the greater the risk:** Dell RM, Adams AL, Green DF, et al. Incidence of atypical nontraumatic diaphyseal fractures of the femur. *J Bone Miner Res.* 2012; 27: 2544–2550.

94 **One out of 1,000:** Schilcher J, Koeppen V, Aspenberg P, et al. Risk of atypical femoral fracture during and after bisphosphonate use. *N Engl J Med.* 2014; 371: 974–976.

94 **No difference in overall fracture risk:** Fraser LA, Vogt KN, Adachi JA, et al. Fracture risk associated with continuation versus discontinuation of bisphosphonates after 5 years of therapy in patients with primary osteoporosis: a systematic review and meta-analysis. *Ther Clin Risk Manag.* 2011; 7: 157–166.

94 **Increased risk of necrosis of the jaw:** Lee SH, Chang SS, Lee M, et al. Risk of osteonecrosis in patients taking bisphosphonates for prevention of osteoporosis: a systematic review and meta-analysis. *Osteoporos Int.* 2014; 25: 1131–1139.

94 **New-onset atrial fibrillation:** Sharma A, Einstein AJ, Vallakati A, et al. Risk of atrial fibrillation with use of oral and intravenous bisphosphonates. *Am J Cardiol.* 2014; 113: 1815–1821.

94 **Seven studies of nearly 20,000 cases:** Andrici J, Tio M, Eslick GD. Meta-analysis: oral bisphosphonates and the risk of esophageal cancer. *Aliment Pharmacol Ther.* 2012; 36: 708–716.

95 **Another analysis found no significant risk:** Wright E, Schofield PT, Molokhia M. Bisphosphonates and evidence for association with esophageal and gastric cancer: a systematic review and meta-analysis. *BMJ Open.* 2015; 5: e007133.

95 **Found to decrease the risk of breast cancer:** Barrett-Connor E, Mosca L, Collins P, et al. Effects of raloxifene on cardiovascular events and breast cancer in postmenopausal women. *N Engl J Med.* 2006; 355: 125–137.

96 **Side effects include headache, muscle and joint pain:** US National Library of Medicine. Medline Plus: Denosumab Injections. July 15, 2015. Accessed at: https://www.nlm.nih.gov/medlineplus/druginfo/meds/a610023.html.

98 **Little evidence that these drugs are helpful or cost-effective:** Schousboe JT, Nyman JA, Kane RL. Cost-effectiveness of alendronate therapy for osteopenic postmenopausal women. *Ann Intern Med.* 2005; 142: 734–741.

Chapter 5: Acid Reflux Disease

99 **Seven out of ten people are taking them:** Forgacs I, Loganayagam A. Overprescribing proton pump inhibitors. *BMJ.* 2008; 336: 2–3.

99 **Nexium was the fourth leading prescription drug:** Brown T. 100 Best selling, most prescribed drugs branded drugs through March. *Medscape Medical News.* May 6, 2015. Available at: http://www.medscape.com/viewarticle/844317.

99 **Nearly one out of five people aged sixty-two and over:** Qato DM, Wilder J, Schumm LP, et al. Changes in prescription and over-the-counter medication and dietary supplement use among older adults in the United States, 2005 vs 2011. *JAMA Intern Med.* 2016; 176: 473–482.

101 **Stop smoking, which relaxes the lower esophageal sphincter:** Kahrilas PJ, Gupta RR. Mechanisms of acid reflux associated with cigarette smoking. *Gut.* 1990; 31: 4–10.

102 **People on the Mediterranean diet:** Mone I, Kraja B, Brugu A. Adherence to a predominantly Mediterranean diet decreases the risk of gastroesophageal reflux disease: a cross-sectional study in a South Eastern European population. *Dis Esophagus.* 2016; 29: 794–800.

102 **People exposed to chronic stress:** Bradley LA, Richter JE, Pulliam TJ, et al. The relationship between stress and symptoms of gastroesophageal reflux: the influence of psychological factors. *Am J Gastroenterol.* 1993; 88: 11–19.

102 **Having psychological problems:** Baker LH, Lieberman D, Oehlke M. Psychological distress in patients with gastroesophageal reflux disease. *Am J Gastroenterol.* 1995; 90: 1797–1803.

102 **Some home remedies that can reduce acid reflux:** http://articles.mercola.com/sites/articles/archive/2014/04/28/acid-reflux-ulcer-treatment.aspx#_edn10.

103 **Acupuncture and Chinese herbs:** Zhang C, Guo L, Guo X, et al. Clinical curative effect of electroacupuncture combined with zhizhukuanzhong capsules for treating gastroesophageal reflux disease. *J Tradit Chin Med.* 2012; 32: 364–371.

103 **People taking PPIs who were still having troublesome symptoms:** Dickman R, Schiff E, Holland A, et al. Clinical trial: acupuncture vs. doubling the proton pump inhibitor dose in refractory heartburn. *Aliment Pharmacol Ther.* 2007; 26: 1333–1344.

104 **Only half of all users were completely free of symptoms:** Kahrilas, PJ. Gastroesophageal reflux disease. *NEJM.* 2008; 359: 1700–1707.

105 **A study in Colorado of almost 6.6 million hospitalized:** Reid M, Keniston A, Heller JC, et al. Inappropriate prescribing of proton pump inhibitors in hospitalized patients. *J Hosp Med.* 2012; 7: 421–425.

106 **Twice the incidence of vitamin B12 deficiency:** Lam JR, Schneider JL, Zhao W, et al. Proton pump inhibitor and histamine 2 receptor antagonist use and vitamin B12 deficiency. *JAMA.* 2013; 310: 2435–2442.

106 **Case reports of patients with severe depression and low vitamin B$_{12}$ levels:** Hanna S, Lachover L, Rajarethinam RP. Vitamin B12 deficiency and depression in the elderly: Review and Case Report. *Prim Care Companion J Clin Psychiatry.* 2009; 11: 269–270.

107 **PPIs can increase the incidence of dementia:** Gomm W, von Holt K, Thomé F, et al. Association of proton pump inhibitors with risk of dementia: a pharmacoepidemiological claims data analysis. *JAMA Neurol.* 2016; 73: 410–416.

107 **10,000 new cases of dementia each year:** Kuller LH. Do proton pump inhibitors increase the risk of dementia? *JAMA Neurol.* 2016; 73: 379–381.

107 **The connection between *C. difficile* and the use of stomach-acid suppressors:** Dial S, Delaney JA, Barkun AN, et al. Use of gastric acid-suppressive agents and the risk of community-acquired *Clostridium difficile*-associated disease. *JAMA.* 2005; 294: 2989–2995.

107 **FDA safety announcement:** U.S. Food and Drug Administration. FDA Drug Safety Communication: *Clostridium difficile*-associated diarrhea can be associated with stomach acid drugs known as proton pump inhibitors (PPIs). http://www.fda.gov/Drugs/DrugSafety/ucm290510.htm.

107 **The results of thirty different studies:** Deshpande A, Pant C, Pasupuleti V, et al. Association between proton pump inhibitor therapy and

Clostridium difficile infection in a meta-analysis. *Clin Gastroenterol Hepatol.* 2012; 10: 225–233.

108 **People taking PPIs have fewer disease-fighting bacteria:** Imhann F, Bonder MJ, Vich Vila A, et al. Proton pump inhibitors affect the gut microbiome. *Gut.* 2016; 65: 740–748.

108 **Nearly two times as likely to develop pneumonia:** Laheij RJ, Sturkenboom MC, Hassing RJ, et al. Risk of community-acquired pneumonia and use of gastric acid-suppressive drugs. *JAMA.* 2004; 292: 1955–1960.

108 **Risk of pneumonia is highest in the first week:** Gulmez SE, Holm A, Frederiksen H, et al. Use of proton pump inhibitors and the risk of community-acquired pneumonia: a population-based case-control study. *Arch Intern Med.* 2007; 167: 950–955.

109 **Meta-analysis of thirty-one different studies:** Eom CS, Jeon CY, Lim JW, et al. Use of acid-suppressive drugs and risk of pneumonia: a systematic review and meta-analysis. *CMAJ.* 2011; 183: 310–319.

109 **The risk of hip fracture in women who had regularly:** Khalili H, Huang ES, Jacobson BC, et al. Use of proton pump inhibitors and risk of hip fracture in relation to dietary and lifestyle factors: a prospective cohort study. *BMJ.* 2012; 344: e372.

109 **Spine, wrist, and forearm fractures:** Gray SL, LaCroix AZ, Larson J, et al. Proton pump inhibitor use, hip fracture, and change in bone mineral density in postmenopausal women: results from the Women's Health Initiative. *Arch Intern Med.* 2010; 170: 765–771.

109 **Patients who take higher doses of PPIs have a greater risk of fractures:** Yang YX, Lewis JD, Epstein S, et al. Long-term proton pump inhibitor therapy and risk of hip fracture. *JAMA.* 2006; 296: 2947–2953.

109 **Those taking them for more than a year:** Targownik LE, Lix LM, Metge CJ, et al. Use of proton pump inhibitors and risk of osteoporosis-related fractures. *CMAJ.* 2008; 179: 319–326.

110 **In a study of more than 10,000 participants followed for up to fourteen years:** Lazarus B, Chen Y, Wilson FP, et al. Proton pump inhibitor use and the risk of chronic kidney disease. *JAMA Intern Med.* 2016; 176: 238–246.

110 **Possible connection between PPIs and heart attacks:** Shah NH, LePendu P, Bauer-Mehren A, Proton pump inhibitor usage and the risk of

myocardial infarction in the general population. *PLoS ONE.* 2015; 10: e0124653.

111 **People who did not have symptoms of acid reflux were randomly divided:** Reimer C, Soundergaard B, Hilsted L, et al. Proton-pump inhibitor therapy induces acid-related symptoms in healthy volunteers after withdrawal of therapy. *Gastroenterology.* 2009; 137: 80–87.

113 **80 million unnecessary prescriptions each year for PPIs:** Katz MH. Failing the acid test: benefits of proton pump inhibitors may not justify the risks for many users. *Arch Intern Med.* 2010; 170: 747–748.

Chapter 6: Depression

115 **7.6 percent of people aged twelve and over:** Pratt LA, Brody DJ. Depression in the U.S. household population, 2009–2012. National Center for Health Statistics. 2014; Data brief no. 172. Accessed at: http://www.cdc.gov/nchs/data/databriefs/db172.htm.

115 **An estimated 8 million doctor visits each year are for depression:** Bishop TF, Ramsay PP, Casalino LP. Care management processes used less often for depression than for other chronic conditions in US primary care practices. *Health Aff.* 2016; 35: 394–400.

115 **Economic burden to the US economy from adults with depression:** Greenberg PE, Fournier A-A, Sisitsky S, et al. The economic burden of adults with major depressive disorder in the United States (2005 and 2010). *J Clin Psychiatry.* 2015; 76: 155–162.

116 **Symptoms can be divided into three main categories:** American Psychiatric Association. *Diagnostic and Statistical Manual of Mental Disorders (DSM–5).* 5th ed. Arlington, VA. 2013.

116 **Suicide rates increased by 24 percent in the fifteen years:** Curtin SC, Warner M, Hedegaard H. Increase in suicide in the United States, 1999–2014. *National Center for Health Statistics.* 2016. Data brief no. 241. Accessed at: http://www.cdc.gov/nchs/products/databriefs/db241.htm.

117 **Suicides . . . related to job, financial, and legal problems:** Hempstead KA, Phillips JA. Rising suicide among adults aged 40–64 years: the role of job and financial circumstances. *Am J Prev Med.* 2015; 48: 491–500.

117 **In a survey of patients with chronic pain:** American Academy of Pain Medicine. AAPM facts and figures on pain. Accessed at: www.painmed.org/patientcenter/facts_on_pain.aspx.

117 **From 8.4 to 11.6 percent of those taking newly-prescribed opioid pain medication:** Scherrer JF, Salas J, Copeland LA, et al. Prescription opioid duration, dose, and increased risk of depression in 3 large patient populations. *Ann Fam Med.* 2016; 14: 54–62.

118 **A nine-item screening instrument that asks about the frequency of symptoms of depression:** Kroenke K, Spitzer RL, Williams JBW. The PHQ–9: Validity of a brief depression severity measure. *J Gen Intern Med.* 2001; 16: 606–613.

119 **Psychotherapy, exercise, acupuncture, and St. John's wort:** Gartlehner G, Gaynes BN, Amick HR, et al. Nonpharmacological versus pharmacological treatments for adult patients with major depressive disorder. Rockville (MD): Agency for Healthcare Research and Quality (US); 2015. Report No.: 15(16)-EHC031-EF.

120 **(CBT) be strongly considered as the first-line treatment for major depression:** Qaseem A, Barry MJ, Devan Kansagara D. Nonpharmacologic versus pharmacologic treatment of adult patients with major depressive disorder: a Clinical Practice Guideline from the American College of Physicians. *Ann Intern Med.* 2016; 164: 350–359.

120 **Cognitive therapy was as effective as switching to a different antidepressant:** Thase ME, Freidman ES, Biggs MM, et al. Cognitive therapy versus medication in augmentation and switch strategies as second-step treatments: a STAR*D report. *Am J Psychiatry.* 2007; 164: 739–752.

121 **Analysis of thirty-seven studies of exercise and depression:** Cooney GM, Dwan K, Greig CA, et al. Exercise for depression. *Cochrane Database Syst Rev.* 2013; 9: CD004366.

121 **Adults aged twenty to forty-five years old who exercised:** Dunn AL, Trivedi MH, Kampert JB, et al. Exercise treatment for depression: efficacy and dose response. *Am J Prev Med.* 2005; 28: 1–8.

121 **Study of 156 adults, 60 to 70 percent of participants in all three treatment groups:** Blumenthal JA, Babyak MA, Moore KA, et al. Effects of exercise training on older patients with major depression. *Arch Intern Med.* 1999; 159: 2349–2356.

122 **Those in the exercise alone group had lower rates of relapse:** Babyak M, Blumenthal JA, Herman S, et al. Exercise treatment for major depression: maintenance of therapeutic benefit at 10 months. *Psychosom Med.* 2000; 62: 633–638.

122 **High intakes of fruit, vegetables, fish, and whole grains have less risk:** Lai JS, Hiles S, Bisquera A, et al. A systematic review and meta-analysis of dietary patterns and depression in community-dwelling adults. *Am J Clin Nutr.* 2014; 99: 181–197.

122 **Low blood levels of folic acid . . . and vitamin B12:** Sanchez-Villegas A, Doreste J, Schlatter J, et al. Association between folate, vitamin B(6) and vitamin B(12) intake and depression in the SUN cohort study. *J Hum Nutr Diet.* 2009; 22: 122–133.

122 **Recent study of nearly 70,000 postmenopausal women:** Gangwisch JE, Hale L, Garcia L, et al. High glycemic index diet as a risk factor for depression: analyses from the Women's Health Initiative. *Am J Clin Nutr.* 2015; 102: 454–463.

122 **The Mediterranean diet decreased the risk of becoming depressed:** Sánchez-Villegas A, Delgado-Rodríguez M, Alonso A, et al. Association of the Mediterranean dietary pattern with the incidence of depression: the Seguimiento Universidad de Navarra/University of Navarra follow-up (SUN) cohort. *Arch Gen Psychiatry.* 2009; 66: 1090–1098.

122 **Diets high in processed foods were associated with increased odds:** Akbaly TN, Brunner EJ, Ferrie JE, et al. Dietary pattern and depressive symptoms in middle age. *Br J Psychiatry.* 2009; 195: 408–413.

122 **Nineteen studies comparing omega-3s with a placebo:** Grosso G, Pajak A, Marventano S, et al. Role of omega-3 fatty acids in the treatment of depressive disorders: a comprehensive meta-analysis of randomized clinical trials. *PLoS One.* 2014; 9: e96905.

123 **Better than placebo in treating depression in a few studies:** Shaw KA, Turner J, Del Mar C. Tryptophan and 5-Hydroxytryptophan for depression. *Cochrane Database System Rev.* 2002; 1: CD003198.

123 **SAMe treatment was as effective as antidepressants:** Freeman MP, Mischoulon D, Tedeschini E, et al. Complementary and alternative medicine for major depressive disorder: a meta-analysis of patient characteristics, placebo-response rates, and treatment outcomes relative to standard antidepressants. *J Clin Psychiatry.* 2010; 71: 682–688.

123 **Vitamin C has been reported to help depressed patients:** Zhang M, Robitaille L, Eintracht S, et al. Vitamin C provision improves mood in acutely hospitalized patients. *Nutrition.* 2011; 27: 530–533.

123 **After eight weeks, light therapy was more effective:** Lam, RW, Levitt AJ, Levitan RD, et al. Efficacy of bright light treatment, fluoxetine, and the combination in patients with nonseasonal major depressive disorder. *JAMA Psychiatry.* 2016; 73: 56–63.

123 **Study of 185 young women in the Pacific Northwest:** Kerr DCR, Zava DT, Piper WT, et al. Associations between vitamin D levels and depressive symptoms in healthy young adult women. *Psychiatr Res.* 2015; 227: 46–51.

124 **Vitamin D was effective in treating people with depression:** Shaffer JA, Edmondson D, Wasson LT, et al. Vitamin D supplementation for depressive symptoms: a systematic review and meta-analysis of randomized controlled trials. *Psychosom Med.* 2014; 76: 190–196.

124 **Vitamin D had an effect that was comparable to that of antidepressant medication:** Spedding S. Vitamin D and depression: a systematic review and meta-analysis comparing studies with and without biological flaws. *Nutrients.* 2014; 6: 1501–1518.

124 **St. John's wort was better than placebo in treating patients with major depression:** Linde K, Berner MM, Kriston L. St John's wort for major depression. *Cochrane Database Syst Rev.* 2008; 4: CD000448.

125 **Acupuncture treatment is comparable to antidepressants:** Zhang ZJ, Chen HY, Yip KC, et al. The effectiveness and safety of acupuncture therapy in depressive disorders: systematic review and meta-analysis. *J Affect Disord.* 2010; 124: 9–21.

125 **Seven hundred and fifty-five patients who were being treated for depression:** MacPherson H, Richmond S, Bland M, et al. Acupuncture and counselling for depression in primary care: a randomised controlled trial. *PloS Med.* 2013; 10: e1001518.

125 **One hundred and thirty-three middle-aged Mexican women with moderate-to-severe depression:** Macias-Cortes EC, Llanes-Gonzalez L, -Aguilar-Faisal L, et al. Individualized homeopathic treatment and -fluoxetine for moderate to severe depression in peri- and postmenopausal women (HOMDEP-MENOP study): a randomized, double-dummy, double-blind, placebo-controlled trial. *PloS One.* 2015; 10: e0127719.

125 **Individualized homeopathic treatment was as effective as fluoxetine:** Adler UC, Paiva NMP, Cesar AT, et al. Homeopathic individualized Q-potencies versus fluoxetine for moderate to severe depression: double-blind,

randomized non-inferiority trial. *Evid Based Complement Alternat Med.* 2011; 2011: 520182.

126 **Study comparing MBCT with maintenance antidepressants:** Kuyken W, Hayes R, Barrett B, et al. Effectiveness and cost-effectiveness of mindfulness-based cognitive therapy compared with maintenance antidepressant treatment in the prevention of depressive relapse or recurrence (PREVENT): a randomised controlled trial. *Lancet.* 2015; 386: 63–73.

126 **Patients using MBCT had a significantly lower risk of recurring depression:** Kuyken W, Warren FC, Taylor RS, et al. Efficacy of Mindfulness-Based Cognitive Therapy in prevention of depressive relapse: an individual patient data meta-analysis from randomized trials. *JAMA Psychiatry.* Published online April 27, 2016. doi:10.1001/jamapsychiatry.2016.0076.

127 **Yoga has been found to be useful in a wide range of mental health disorders:** Balasubramaniam M, Telles S, Doraiswamy PM. Yoga on our minds: a systematic review of yoga for neuropsychiatric disorders. *Front Psychiatry.* 2012; 3: 117.

127 **Massage therapy helps alleviate symptoms of depression:** Hou WH, Chiang PT, Hsu TY, et al. Treatment effects of massage therapy in depressed people: a meta-analysis. *J Clin Psychiatry.* 2010; 71: 894–901.

127 **Studies of biofeedback:** Siepmann M, Aykac V, Unterdorfer J, et al. A pilot study on the effects of heart rate variability biofeedback in patients with depression and in healthy subjects. *Appl Psychophysiol Biofeedback.* 2008; 33: 195–201.

128 **Nearly 9 percent from 2007 to 2010:** Centers for Disease Control and Prevention. Health, United States, 2012. Table 92. Accessed at http://www.cdc.gov/nchs/data/hus/2012/092.pdf.

128 **A Mayo Clinic survey found that more than 12 percent of people:** Zhong W, Maradit-Kremers H, St. Sauver JL, et al. Age and sex patterns of drug prescribing in a defined American population. *Mayo Clin Proc.* 2013; 88: 697–707.

129 **Only 55.2 percent of prescriptions for antidepressants by primary care providers:** Wong J, Motulsky A, Eguale T, et al. Treatment indications for antidepressants prescribed in primary care in Quebec, Canada, 2006–2015. *JAMA.* 2016; 315: 2230–2232.

129 **GlaxoSmithKline was fined $3 billion for promoting Paxil to children:** Neville, S. GlaxoSmithKline fined $3bn after bribing doctors to increase drugs sales. *The Guardian*. July 3, 2012. Accessed at: https://www.theguardian.com/business/2012/jul/03/glaxosmithkline-fined-bribing-doctors-pharmaceuticals.

129 **Meta-analysis of data from six different studies:** Fournier JC, DeRubeis RJ, Hollon SD, et al. Antidepressant drug effects and depression severity: a patient-level meta-analysis. *JAMA*. 2010; 303: 47–53.

130 **The placebo response activates natural opioids in the body:** Peciña M, Bohnert ASB, Sikora M, et al. Association between placebo-activated neural systems and antidepressant responses: neurochemistry of placebo effects in major depression. *JAMA Psychiatry*. 2015; 72: 1087–1094.

130 **For every seven to eight people treated with selective serotonin reuptake inhibitors:** Arrol B, Elley CR, Fishman T, et al. Antidepressants versus placebo for depression in primary care. *Cochrane Database Syst Rev*. 2009; 3: CD007954.

130 **The effect of antidepressants is small and becomes clinically significant:** Kirsch I, Deacon BJ, Huedo-Medina TB, et al. Initial severity and antidepressant benefits: a meta-analysis of data submitted to the Food and Drug Administration. *PloS Med*. 2008; 5: e45.

130 **Only one-third of participants became symptom-free:** National Institute of Mental Health. Questions and answers about the NIMH sequenced treatment alternatives to relieve depression (STAR*D) study—all medication levels. 2006. Accessed at: http://www.nimh.nih.gov/funding/clinical-research/practical/stard/allmedicationlevels.shtml.

130 **Analysis of seventy-four studies registered with the FDA:** Turner EH, Matthews AM, Linardatos E, et al. Selective publication of antidepressant trials and its influence on apparent efficacy. *NEJM*. 2008; 358: 252–260

131 **There is no conclusive evidence that low serotonin in the brain is associated with depression:** Lacasse JR, Leo J. Serotonin and depression: a disconnect between the advertisements and the scientific literature. *PLoS Med*. 2005; 2: e392.

132 **The concept that depression is the result of low serotonin levels is a myth:** Healy D. Serotonin and depression. *BMJ*. 2015; 350: h1771.

132 **TCAs have been linked to an increased risk of dementia:** Gray SL, Anderson ML, Dublin S, et al. Cumulative use of strong anticholinergics and incident dementia. *JAMA Intern Med.* 2015; 175: 401–407.

133 **British study of 160,000 patients taking tricyclic or SSRI antidepressants:** Jick H, Kaye JA, Jick SS. Antidepressants and the risk of suicidal behaviors. *JAMA.* 2004; 292: 338–343.

134 **Studies have not shown any significant differences between SSRIs and SNRIs:** Thase ME. Are SNRIs more effective than SSRIs? A review of the current state of the controversy. *Psychopharmacol Bull.* 2008; 41: 58–85.

134 **Sixteen to 29 percent of people who start therapy with antidepressants stop them:** O'Connor EA, Whitlock EP, Gaynes B, et al. Screening for depression in adults and older adults in primary care: an updated systematic review. Agency for Healthcare Research and Quality. 2009. Accessed at: http://www.ncbi.nlm.nih.gov/books/NBK36400/.

135 **Twice as many suicide attempts in those taking SSRIs:** Fergusson D, Doucette S, Glass KC, et al. Association between suicide attempts and selective serotonin reuptake inhibitors: systematic review of randomised controlled trials. *BMJ.* 2005; 330: 396.

135 **In 2007, the FDA ordered a "black box" warning:** United States Food and Drug Administration. Antidepressant Use in Children, Adolescents, and Adults. May 2, 2007. Accessed at: http://www.fda.gov/Drugs /DrugSafety/InformationbyDrugClass/UCM096273.

135 **58 percent increased risk of suicidal thoughts and behavior:** Hetrick SE, McKenzie JE, Cox GR, et al. Newer generation antidepressants for depressive disorders in children and adolescents. *Cochrane Database Syst Rev.* 2012; 11: CD004851.

135 **Those taking higher doses have a greater risk:** Miller M, Swanson SA, Azrael D, et al. Antidepressant dose, age, and the risk of deliberate self-harm. *JAMA Intern Med.* 2014; 174: 899.

135 **Twice the risk of suicidal and aggressive behavior in children and adolescents:** Sharma T, Guski LS, Freund N, et al. Suicidality and aggression during antidepressant treatment: systematic review and meta-analyses based on clinical study reports. *BMJ.* 2016; 352: i65.

136 **SSRI antidepressants were more than eight times as likely to be associated with violent behavior:** Moore TJ, Glenmullen J, Furberg CD.

Prescription drugs associated with reports of violence towards others. *PLoS One.* 2010; 5: e15337.

136 **Legal defense in several cases involving homicide:** Healy D, Herxheimer A, Menkes DB. Antidepressants and violence: problems at the interface of medicine and law. *PLoS Med.* 2006; 3: e372.

136 **Forty-three percent increased rate of convictions for violent crimes:** Molero Y, Lichtenstein P, Zetterqvist J, et al. Selective serotonin reuptake inhibitors and violent crime: a cohort study. *PLoS Med.* 2015; 12: e1001875.

136 **Repeated doses of a common antidepressant stimulated parts of the brain:** Ricci LA, Melloni RH. Repeated fluoxetine administration during adolescence stimulates aggressive behavior and alters serotonin and vasopressin neural development in hamsters. *Behav Neurosci.* 2013; 126: 640–653.

136 **More than one-and-a-half times the risk of developing upper gastrointestinal bleeding:** Jiang HY, Chen HZ, Hu XJ, et al. Use of selective serotonin reuptake inhibitors and risk of upper gastrointestinal bleeding: a systematic review and meta-analysis. *Clin Gastroenterol Hepatol.* 2015; 13: 42–50e43.

136 **Especially when combined with nonsteroidal anti-inflammatory drugs:** Anglin R, Yuan Y, Moayyedi P, et al. Risk of upper gastrointestinal bleeding with selective serotonin reuptake inhibitors with or without concurrent nonsteroidal anti-inflammatory use: a systematic review and meta-analysis. *Am J Gastroenterol.* 2014; 109: 811–819.

136 **A recent meta-analysis reported a 40 percent increase in strokes:** Shin D, Oh YH, Eom C-S, et al. Use of selective serotonin reuptake inhibitors and risk of stroke: a systematic review and meta-analysis. *J Neurol.* 2014; 261: 686–695.

136 **Twice as likely to experience microbleeds:** Akoudad S, Aarts N, Roordam R, et al. Antidepressant use is associated with an increased risk of developing microbleeds. *Stroke.* 2016; 47: 251–254.

136 **Unnoticed strokes in the brain that have been associated with mental impairment:** Martinez-Ramirez S, Greenberg SM, Viswanathan A, et al. Cerebral microbleeds: overview and implications in cognitive impairment. *Alzheimers Res Ther.* 2014; 6: 33.

136 **A potentially life-threatening problem for those taking SSRIs is hypo-natremia:** Jacob S, Spinler SA. Hyponatremia associated with selective serotonin-reuptake inhibitors in older adults. *Ann Pharmacother.* 2006; 40: 1618–1622.

137 **Other classes of antidepressants have also been found to cause hypo-natremia:** De Picker L, Van Den Eede F, Dumont G, et al. Antidepressants and the risk of hyponatremia: a class-by-class review of literature. *Psychosomatics.* 2014; 55: 536–547.

137 **People who are taking antidepressants of all kinds:** Bhattacharjee S, Bhattacharya R, Kelley GA. Antidepressant use and new-onset diabetes: a systematic review and meta-analysis. *Diabetes Metab Res Rev.* 2013; 29: 273–284.

137 **A study of nearly 36,000 African American women followed for twelve years:** Vimalananda VG, Palmer JR, Gerlovin H, et al. Depressive symptoms, antidepressant use, and the incidence of diabetes in the Black Women's Health Study. *Diabetes Care.* 2014; 37: 2211–2217.

137 **The risk of death from any cause was 54 percent higher:** Coupland C, Dhiman C, Arthur A, et al. Antidepressant use and risk of adverse outcomes in older people: population based cohort study. *BMJ.* 2011; 343: d4551.

138 **The FDA issued a warning that SSRIs may be associated with this syndrome:** U.S. Food and Drug Administration. Selective serotonin reuptake inhibitor (SSRI) antidepressant use during pregnancy and reports of a rare heart and lung condition in newborn babies. Dec 14, 2011. Accessed at: http://www.fda.gov/Drugs/DrugSafety/ucm283375.htm.

138 **One case of PPHN is likely to occur for every 286 to 351 women:** Grigoriadis S, VonderPorten ES, Mamisashvili L, et al. Prenatal exposure to antidepressants and persistent pulmonary hypertension of the newborn: systematic review and meta-analysis. *BMJ.* 2014; 348: f6932.

138 **Researchers analyzed data from more than 145,000 children born in Quebec:** Boukhris T, Sheehy O, Mottron L, et al. Antidepressant use during pregnancy and the risk of autism spectrum disorder in children. *JAMA Pediatr.* 2016; 170: 117–124.

138 **Boys whose mothers took SSRIs during pregnancy were nearly three times as likely:** Harrington RA, Lee L-C, Crum RM, et al. Prenatal SSRI use and offspring with autism spectrum disorder or developmental delay. *Pediatrics.* 2014; 133: e1241–e1248.

139 **Withdrawal symptoms occur in about 20 percent of people:** Warner CH, Bobo W, Warner C, et al. Antidepressant discontinuation syndrome. *Am Fam Physician.* 2006; 74: 449–456.

139 **Symptoms such as anxiety, depression, fatigue, flulike symptoms, muscle spasms, tremors:** Fava GA, Gatti A, Belaise C, et al. Withdrawal symptoms after selective serotonin reuptake inhibitor discontinuation: a systematic review. *Psychother Psychosom.* 2015; 84: 72–81.

Chapter 7: Chronic Pain: Back, Neck, and Osteoarthritic

144 **Chronic pain affects at least 100 million Americans:** Institute of Medicine. *Relieving Pain in America: A Blueprint for Transforming Prevention, Care, Education and Research.* The National Academies Press, 2011.

144 **More than 28 percent of US adults reported having low back pain:** Centers for Disease Control and Prevention. Health United States: 2015. Table 41. Accessed at: http://www.cdc.gov/nchs/data/hus/2015/041.pdf.

145 **In 2016, there were more than:** National Institute of Drug Abuse. Overdose death rates. Accessed at: https://www.drugabuse.gov/related-topics /trends-statistics/overdose-death-rates

146 **Smoking has been linked to an increase in back pain:** Goldberg MS, Scott SC, Mayo NF. A review of the association between cigarette smoking and the development of nonspecific back pain and related outcomes. *Spine.* 2000; 25: 995–1014.

146 **Patients with new-onset low back pain remain active and use self-care measures:** Chou R, Qaseem A, Snow V, et al. Diagnosis and treatment of low back pain: a joint clinical practice guideline from the American College of Physicians and the American Pain Society. *Ann Intern Med.* 2007; 147: 478–491.

146 **Nonpharmacologic treatments:** Chou R, Huffman LH. Nonpharmacologic therapies for acute and chronic low back pain: a review of the evidence for an American Pain Society/American College of Physicians clinical practice guideline. *Ann Intern Med.* 2007; 147: 492–504.

146 **A survey of general practice physicians reported that more than 25 percent of them:** Williams CM, Maher CG, Hancock MJ. Low back pain and best practice care: A survey of general practice physicians. *Arch Intern Med.* 2010; 170: 271–277.

147 **A study of 32,070 patients with low back pain:** Fritz JM, Childs JD, Wainner RS, et al. Primary care referral of patients with low back pain to physical therapy: impact on future health care utilization and costs. *Spine.* 2012; 37: 2114–2121.

147 **Analysis of more than 750,000 patients with low back pain in the US military:** Childs JD, Fritz JM, Wu SS, et al. Implications of early and guideline adherent physical therapy for low back pain on utilization and costs. *BMC Health Serv Res.* 2015; 15: 150.

147 **Seventy-four percent of people who used alternative therapies:** Kanodia AK, Legedza AT, Davis RB, et al. Perceived benefit of Complementary and Alternative Medicine (CAM) for back pain: a national survey. *J Am Board Fam Med.* 2010; 23: 354–362.

147 **Spinal manipulation is effective for acute, subacute, and chronic low back pain:** Bronfort G, Haas M, Evans R, et al. Effectiveness of manual therapies: the UK evidence report. *Chiropr Osteopat.* 2010; 18: 3.

147 **Twenty-six trials of spinal manipulation in patients who had suffered from low back pain:** Rubinstein SM, van Middelkoop M, Assendelft WJ, et al. Spinal manipulative therapy for chronic low-back pain. *Cochrane Database of Syst Rev.* 2011; 2: CD008112.

148 **Those receiving massage therapy used less medication:** Cherkin DC, Sherman KJ, Kahn J, et al. A comparison of the effects of 2 types of massage and usual care on chronic low back pain: a randomized, controlled trial. *Ann Intern Med.* 2011; 155: 1–9.

148 **Exercise reduces low back pain and improves the long-term functioning:** van-Middelkoop M, Rubinstein SM, Verhagen AP, et al. Exercise therapy for chronic nonspecific low-back pain. *Best Pract Res Clin Rheumatol.* 2010; 24: 193–204.

149 **Exercise also is effective in preventing low back pain:** Steffens D, Maher CD, Pereira LSM, et al. Prevention of low back pain: a systematic review and meta-analysis. *JAMA Intern Med.* 2016; 176: 199–208.

149 **Those taking yoga classes over a twelve-week period:** Tilbrook HE, Cox H, Hewitt CE, et al. Yoga for chronic low back pain: a randomized trial. *Ann Intern Med.* 2011; 155: 569–578.

149 **Yoga and stretching exercises led by a physical therapist:** Sherman KJ, Cherkin DC, Wellman RD, et al. A randomized trial comparing yoga,

stretching, and a self-care book for chronic low back pain. *Arch Intern Med.* 2011; 171: 2019–2026.

149 **Acupuncture was effective for several types of chronic pain:** Vickers AJ, Cronin AM, Maschino AC, et al. Acupuncture for chronic pain: individual patient data meta-analysis. *Arch Intern Med.* 2012; 172: 1444–1453.

149 **Acupuncture is cost-effective and better than standard care:** Cummings M. Modellvorhaben Akupunktur—a summary of the ART, ARC and GERAC trials. *Acupunct Med.* 2009; 27: 26–30.

150 **One hundred twenty-nine adults who had suffered from low back pain:** Witt CM, Ludtke R, Baur R, et al. Homeopathic treatment of patients with chronic low back pain: A prospective observational study with 2 years' follow-up. *Clin J Pain.* 2009; 25: 334–339.

150 **Twenty-three studies of over 6,000 people with chronic low back pain:** Richmond H, Hall AM, Copsey B, et al. The Effectiveness of Cognitive Behavioural Treatment for Non-Specific Low Back Pain: A Systematic Review and Meta-Analysis. *PloS One.* 2015; 10: e0134192.

150 **Better than usual care in a study that evaluated pain and functioning:** Cherkin DC, Sherman KJ, Balderson BH, et al. Effect of mindfulness-based stress reduction vs cognitive behavioral therapy or usual care on back pain and functional limitations in adults with chronic low back pain: a randomized clinical trial. *JAMA.* 2016; 315: 1240–1249.

151 **15 percent of adults reported having had neck pain:** Centers for Disease Control and Prevention. Health United States: 2015. Table 41. Accessed at: http://www.cdc.gov/nchs/data/hus/2015/041.pdf.

152 **Evaluated acupuncture and the Alexander Technique:** MacPherson H, Tilbrook H, Richmond S, et al. Alexander Technique lessons or acupuncture sessions for persons with chronic neck pain: a randomized trial. *Ann Intern Med.* 2015; 163: 653–662.

152 **Degenerative joint disease, affects over 30 million:** Centers for Disease Control and Prevention. Osteoarthritis Fact Sheet. Accessed at: www.cdc .gov/arthritis/basics/osteoarthritis.htm.

152 **More than one-third of the US population aged sixty or older:** Lawrence RC, Felson DT, Helmick CG, et al. Estimates of the prevalence of arthritis and other rheumatic conditions in the United States. Part II. *Arthritis Rheum.* 2008; 58: 26–35.

153 **Aerobic, muscle strengthening, water, and tai chi exercises all helped improve:** Bennell KL, Hinman RS. A review of the clinical evidence for exercise in osteoarthritis of the hip and knee. *J Sci Med Sport.* 2011; 14: 4–9.

154 **A meta-analysis of ninety-one different studies of people with knee OA:** Rogers MR, Semple S. Exercise as an intervention for osteoarthritis of the knee: A review of the literature. *Int Sportmed J.* 2012; 14: 260–293.

154 **Dropping just ten to fifteen pounds can alleviate pain:** Christensen R, Bartels EM, Astrup A, et al. Effect of weight reduction in obese patients diagnosed with knee osteoarthritis: a systematic review and meta-analysis/ *Ann Rheum* Dis. 2007; 66: 433–439.

154 **For every pound lost, four pounds less pressure was exerted:** Messier SP, Gutekunst DJ, Davis C, et al. Weight loss reduces knee-joint loads in overweight and obese older adults with knee osteoarthritis. *Arthritis Rheum.* 2005; 52: 2026–2032.

155 **Direct relationship between weight gain or loss . . . the actual amount of cartilage:** Teichtahl AJ, Wlukal AE, Tanamus SK, et al. Weight change and change in tibial cartilage volume and symptoms in obese adults. *Ann Rheum Dis.* 2015; 74: 1024–1029.

155 **A study of 454 overweight or obese sedentary people:** Messier SP, Mihalko SL, Legault C, et al. Effects of intensive diet and exercise on knee joint loads, inflammation, and clinical outcomes among overweight and obese adults with knee osteoarthritis. *JAMA.* 2013; 310: 1263–1273.

155 **Diets high in fiber, healthy oils (omega-3 fatty acids):** Tick H. Nutrition and pain. *Phys Med Rehabil Clin N Am.* 2015; 26: 309–320.

156 **Those receiving 2 grams per day of curcumin extract for six weeks:** Kuptniratsaikul V, Thanakhumtorn S, Chinswangwatanakul P, et al. Efficacy and safety of Curcuma domestic extracts in patients with knee osteoarthritis. *J Altern Complement Med.* 2009; 15: 891–897.

156 **Ginger extract can significantly reduce knee pain:** Altman RD, Marcussen KC. Effects of a ginger extract on knee pain in patients with osteoarthritis. *Arthritis Rheum.* 2001; 44: 2531–2538.

156 **Supplementation with omega-3s for three to four months:** Goldberg RJ, Katz J. A meta-analysis of the analgesic effects of omega-3 polyunsaturated fatty acid supplementation for inflammatory joint pain. *Pain.* 2007; 129: 210–223.

156 **Preliminary evidence that omega-3s also can be beneficial:** Boe C, Vangsness CT. Fish oil and osteoarthritis: current evidence. *Am J Orthop.* 2015; 44: 302–305.

156 **2016 meta-analysis found that for people with OA, practicing tai chi:** Kong LJ, Lauche R, Klose P, et al. Tai Chi for chronic pain conditions: a systematic review and meta-analysis of randomized controlled trials. *Sci Rep.* 2016; 6: 25325.

156 **204 patients with knee OA who were randomized to receive either tai chi:** Wang C, Schmid CH, Iversen MD, et al. Comparative effectiveness of Tai chi versus physical therapy for knee osteoarthritis: a randomized trial. *Ann Intern Med.* doi:10.7326/M15-2143.

157 **2006 study funded by the National Institutes of Health (NIH):** Clegg DO, Reda DJ, Harris CL, et al. Glucosamine, chondroitin sulfate, and the two in combination for painful knee osteoarthritis. *N Engl J Med.* 2006; 354: 795–808.

157 **Significant reduction in joint space narrowing:** Fransen M, Agaliotis M, Nairn L, et al. Glucosamine and chondroitin for knee osteoarthritis: a double-blind randomised placebo-controlled clinical trial evaluating single and combination regimens. *Ann Rheum Dis.* 2015; 74: 851–858.

157 **A product containing glucosamine (500 milligrams) and chondroitin:** Hochberg MC, Martel-Pelletier J, Monfort J, et al. Combined chondroitin sulfate and glucosamine for painful knee osteoarthritis: a multicentre, randomised, double-blind, non-inferiority trial versus celecoxib. *Ann Rheum Dis.* 2016; 75: 37–44.

160 **Ineffective for the treatment of low back pain and provides only minimal short-term benefit:** Machado GC, Maher CG, Ferriera PH, et al. Efficacy and safety of paracetamol for spinal pain and osteoarthritis: systematic review and meta-analysis of randomised placebo controlled trials. *BMJ.* 2015; 350: h1225.

160 **Acetaminophen was no better than placebo for pain relief:** Saragiotto BT, Machado GC, Ferreira ML, et al. Paracetamol for low back pain. *Cochrane Database Syst Rev.* 2016; 6: CD012230.

160 **Liver damage when taken for only fourteen days:** Watkins PB, Kaplowitz N, Slatatery JT, et al. Aminotransferase elevations in healthy adults receiving 4 grams of acetaminophen daily: a randomized controlled trial. *JAMA.* 2006; 296: 87–93.

160 **Acetaminophen causes almost half of all acute liver failure cases in the United States:** Lee WM. Recent developments in acute liver failure. *Best Pract Res Clin Gastroenterol.* 2012; 26: 3–16.

160 **Acetaminophen overdose is the leading reason for calls to poison control centers:** Mowry JB, Spyker DA, Brooks DE, et al. 2014 Annual Report of the American Association of Poison Control Centers' National Poison Data System (NPDS): 32nd Annual Report. *Clin Toxicol.* 2015; 10: 962–1147.

160 **More than 33,000 hospitalizations, and an estimated 300 deaths:** Miller TC, Gerth J. Behind the numbers. September 20, 2013. Accessed at: https://www.propublica.org/article/tylenol-mcneil-fda-behind-the-numbers.

160 **Review of the long-term effects of acetaminophen reported evidence:** Roberts E, Nunes VD, Buckner S, et al. Paracetamol: not as safe as we thought? A systematic literature review of observational studies. *Ann Rheum Dis.* 2016; 75: 552–559.

161 **30 million people use NSAIDs every day, and they account for 60 percent:** Sostres C, Gargallo CJ, Lanas A. Nonsteroidal anti-inflammatory drugs and upper and lower gastrointestinal mucosal damage. *Arthritis Res Ther.* 2013; 15: S3.

161 **Seventeen different placebo-controlled studies of people with chronic knee pain:** Smith SR, Deshpande BR, Collins JE, et al. Comparative pain reduction of oral nonsteroidal anti-inflammatory drugs and opioids for knee osteoarthritis: systematic analytic review. *Osteoarthritis Cartilage.* 2016; 24: 962–972.

161 **More than 100,000 hospital admissions annually in the United States:** Fine M. Quantifying the impact of NSAID-associated adverse events. *Am J Manag Care.* 2013; 19: S267–S272.

162 **NSAIDs have been associated with a two- to threefold increased risk of heart attacks and strokes:** Trelle S, Reichenbach S, Wandel S, et al. Cardiovascular safety of nonsteroidal anti-inflammatory drugs: network meta-analysis. *BMJ.* 2011; 342: c7086.

162 **FDA issued a safety announcement in July 2015:** US Food and Drug Administration. FDA Drug Safety Communication: FDA strengthens warning that non-aspirin nonsteroidal anti-inflammatory drugs (NSAIDs) can cause heart attacks or strokes. July 9, 2015. Accessed at: http://www.fda.gov/Drugs/DrugSafety/ucm451800.htm.

162 **Risk of heart attack is highest in the first month of taking NSAIDs:** Bally M, Dendukuri A, Rich B, et al. Risk of acute myocardial infarction with NSAIDs in real world use: bayesian meta-analysis of individual patient data. *BMJ.* 2017: 357; j1909.

162 **Combining NSAIDs with antidepressants increases the risk of bleeding:** Shin J-Y, Park, M-J, Lee SH, et al. Risk of intracranial haemorrhage in antidepressant users with concurrent use of non-steroidal anti-inflammatory drugs: nationwide propensity score matched study. *BMJ.* 2015; 351: h3517.

163 **These topical agents are as effective as oral NSAIDs when compared to a placebo:** Simon LS, Grierson LM, Naseer Z, et al. Efficacy and safety of topical diclofenac containing dimethyl sulfoxide (DMSO) compared with those of topical placebo, DMSO vehicle and oral diclofenac for knee osteoarthritis. *Pain.* 2009; 143: 238–245.

164 **COX-2 inhibitors carry a higher risk of heart attacks and strokes:** Coxib and traditional NSAID Trialists' (CNT) Collaboration. Vascular and upper gastrointestinal effects of non-steroidal anti-inflammatory drugs: meta-analyses of individual participant data from randomised trials. *Lancet.* 2013; 382: 769–779.

164 **Study comparing steroid with saline (a sterile salt solution) injections:** McAlindon TE, LaValley MP, Harvey WF. Effect of intra-articular triamcinolone vs saline on knee cartilage volume and pain in patients with knee osteoarthritis. *JAMA.* 2017; 317: 1967–1975.

165 **There is little proof of their safety and effectiveness:** Kissin I. Long-term opioid treatment of chronic nonmalignant pain: unproven efficacy and neglected safety? *J Pain Res.* 2013; 6: 513–529.

165 **Opioids are no better than NSAIDs in relieving pain:** Chaparro LE, Furlan AD, Deshpande A, et al. Opioids compared to placebo or other treatments for chronic low-back pain. *Cochrane Database Syst Rev.* 2013; 8: CD004959.

165 **The effectiveness of opioids for chronic noncancer pain:** Furlan AD, Sandoval JA, Mailis-Gagnon A, et al. Opioids for chronic noncancer pain: a meta-analysis of effectiveness and side effects. *CMAJ.* 2006; 174: 1589–1594.

165 **Meta-analysis of opioids for knee and hip pain:** da Costa BR, Nuesch E, Kasteler R, et al. Oral or transdermal opioids for osteoarthritis of the knee or hip. *Cochrane Database Syst Rev.* 2014; 9: CD003115.

166 **Opioids can also increase the risk of depression:** Scherrer JF, Salas J, Copeland LA, et al. Prescription opioid duration, dose, and increased risk of depression in 3 large patient populations. *Ann Fam Med.* 2016; 14: 54–62.

166 **Taking opioids with antidepressants increases the risk of serotonin syndrome:** U.S. Food and Drug Administration. FDA Drug Safety Communication: FDA warns about several safety issues with opioid pain medicines; requires label changes. March 22, 2016. Accessed at: http://www.fda .gov/Drugs/DrugSafety/ucm489676.htm.

166 **More than four million people use painkillers for nonmedical reasons:** National Safety Council. Painkillers at root of prescription drug overdose epidemic. 2016. Accessed at: http://www.nsc.org/learn/NSC-Initiatives/Pages /prescription-painkiller-epidemic.aspx?utm_medium=%28none%29&utm _source=%28direct%29&utm_campaign=rxpainkillers.

166 **CDC has issued new guidelines to doctors for opioid prescribing:** Dowell D, Haegerich TM, Chou R. CDC Guideline for Prescribing Opioids for Chronic Pain—United States, 2016. *JAMA.* 2016; 315: 1624–1645.

169 **First line of treatment for chronic pain by NICE:** National Institute for Health and Care Excellence. Osteoarthritis: care and management. February, 2014. Accessed at: https://www.nice.org.uk/guidance/cg177 /chapter/1 recommendations.

Chapter 8: High Blood Pressure

171 **75 million adults in the United States:** Merai R, Siegel C, Rakotz M, et al. CDC Grand Rounds: A public health approach to detect and control hypertension. *MMR Morb Mortal Wkly Rep.* 2016; 65: 1261–1264.

171 **46 billion in health-care services:** Mozzafarian D, Benjamin EJ, Go AS, et al. Heart disease and stroke statistics—2015 update: a report from the American Heart Association. *Circulation.* 2015; e29–322.

172 **Expert guidelines recommend that blood pressure be taken after sitting quietly for five to ten minutes:** Final recommendation statement: high blood pressure in adults: screening. U.S. Preventive Services Task Force. November 2015. Accessed at: http://www.uspreventiveser vicestaskforce.org/Page/Document/RecommendationStatementFinal /high-blood-pressure-in-adults-screening.

172 **15 to 30 percent of people diagnosed with hypertension:** Piper MA, Evans CV, Burda BU, et al. Screening for high blood pressure in adults: a systematic

evidence review for the U.S. Preventive Services Task Force. 2014. Agency for Healthcare Research and Quality Publication No.13-05194-EF-1.

174 **Conflicts of interest from seventeen different pharmaceutical and device manufacturers:** James PA, Oparil S, Carter BL, et al. 2014 evidence-based guideline for the management of high blood pressure in adults. *JAMA.* 2014; 311: 507–520.

174 **According to the guidelines of several expert groups:** Gauer R, Larocque J. JNC 8: relaxing the standards. *Am Fam Physician.* 2014; 90: 449–452.

174 **Co-chair of a group issuing guidelines:** O'Riordan M. New European hypertension guidelines released: goal is less than 140 mmHg for all. *Medscape Medical News.* June 15, 2013. Accessed at: http://www.medscape .com/viewarticle/806367?nlid=31771_1821&src=wnl_edit_dai l&uac=26118EV.

174 **A review of several studies of otherwise healthy people:** Diao D, Wright JM, Cundiff DK, et al. Pharmacotherapy for mild hypertension. *Cochrane Database Syst Rev.* 2012; 8: CD006742.

174 **2014 editorial in the highly regarded *British Medical Journal*:** Martin SA, Boucher M, Wright JM, et al. Mild hypertension in people at low risk. *BMJ.* 2014; 349: g5432.

175 **2014 hypertension guidelines:** James PA, Oparil S, Carter BL, et al. 2014 evidence-based guideline for the management of high blood-pressure in adults. *JAMA.* 2014; 311: 507–520.

175 **Previous guidelines, published in 2004:** Joint National Committee on Prevention, Evaluation, and Treatment of High Blood Pressure. *The Seventh Report of the Joint National Committee on Prevention, Detection, Evaluation, and Treatment of High Blood Pressure.* Bethesda, MD. US Dept of Health and Human Services 2004; NIH publication 04–5230.

175 **Expert panel made up mostly of nutritionists:** Eckel RH, Jakicic JM, Ard JD, et al. 2013 AHA/ACC guideline on lifestyle management to reduce cardiovascular risk. *Circulation.* 2014; 129: S76–S99.

176 **DASH information:** National Heart, Lung, and Blood Institute. Description of DASH eating plan. September 16, 2015. Accessed at: https://www .nhlbi.nih.gov/health/health-topics/topics/dash.

176 **The ability of the DASH diet to lower blood pressure:** Blumenthal JA, Babyak MA, Hinderliter A, et al. Effects of the DASH diet alone and in combination with exercise and weight loss on blood pressure and

cardiovascular biomarkers in men and women with high blood pressure. *Arch of Intern Med.* 2010; 170: 126.

177 **Recent survey of common processed foods:** Jacobson M, Havas S, McCarter R. Changes in sodium levels in processed and restaurant foods, 2005 to 2011. *JAMA Intern Med.* 2013; 173: 1285–1291.

178 **Study of twenty-six chain sit-down restaurants:** Scourboutakos MJ, Semnani-Azad Z, L'Abbe MR. Restaurant meals: almost a full day's worth of calories, fats, and sodium. *JAMA Intern Med.* 2013; 173: 1373–1374.

179 **A meta-analysis of twenty-eight studies of tai chi:** Harrison L. Tai Chi resembles drugs, aerobics in blood pressure lowering. *Medscape Medical News.* June 1, 2016. Accessed at: http://www.medscape.com/viewarticle/864177.

179 **Electroacupuncture . . . was effective in lowering blood pressure:** Peng L, Tjen-A-Looi SC, Ling C, et al. Long-lasting reduction of blood pressure by electroacupuncture in patients with hypertension: randomized controlled trial. *Med Acupunct.* 2015; 27: 253–266.

179 **Acupuncture is effective in lowering blood pressure:** Flachskampf FA, Gallasch J, Gefeller O, et al. Randomized trial of acupuncture to lower blood pressure. *Circulation.* 2007; 115: 3121–3129.

187 **Twelve-year study of more than 3,000 African Americans:** Liu H, Gao SJ, Hall KS, et al. Optimal blood pressure for cognitive function: findings from an elderly African-American cohort study. *J Am Geriatr Soc.* 2013; 61: 875–881.

187 **Patients who already had dementia or mild cognitive impairment** Mossello E, Pieraccioli M, Nesti N, et al. Effects of low blood pressure in cognitively impaired elderly patients treated with antihypertensive drugs. *JAMA Intern Med.* 2015; 175: 578–585.

188 **Italian study of people aged seventy-five and older:** Ogliari G, Sabayan B, Mari D, et al. Age and functional status–dependent association between blood pressure and cognition: The Milan Geriatrics 75+ Cohort Study. *J Am Geriatr Soc.* 2015; 63: 1741.

188 **5,000 adults over age seventy:** Tinetti ME, Han L, Lee DSH. Antihypertensive medications and serious fall injuries in a nationally representative sample of older adults. *JAMA Intern Med.* 2014; 174: 588–595.

188 **Veterans ages forty-five to eighty-five:** Tringali S, Oberer CW, Huang J. Low diastolic blood pressure as a risk for all-cause mortality in VA Patients. *Int J Hypertens.* 2013; 2013: 178780.

188 **Frail nursing home residents:** Benetos A, Labat C, Rossignol P, et al. Treatment with multiple blood pressure medications, achieved blood pressure, and mortality in older nursing home residents: The PARTAGE study. *JAMA Intern Med.* 2015; 175: 989–995.

189 **Review of nineteen different studies:** Xie X, Atkins E, Lv J, et al. Effects of intensive blood pressure lowering on cardiovascular and renal outcomes: updated systematic review and meta-analysis. *Lancet.* 2016; 387: 435–443.

189 **The SPRINT study:** The SPRINT research group. A randomized trial of intensive versus standard blood-pressure control. *N Engl J Med.* 2015; 373: 2103–2116.

190 **400,000 members of a large health maintenance organization:** Sim JJ, Shi J, Kovesdy CP, et al. Impact of achieved blood pressures on mortality risk and end-stage renal disease among a large, diverse hypertension population. *J Am Coll Cardiol.* 2014; 64: 588–597.

Chapter 9: Type 2 Diabetes

193 **According to official government reports:** Centers for Disease Control and Prevention. *National Diabetes Statistics Report: Estimates of Diabetes and Its Burden in the United States, 2017.* Accessed at https://www.cdc.gov/diabetes/pdfs/data/statistics/national-diabetes-statistics-report.pdf.

195 **Lifestyle interventions such as a healthy diet:** Selph S, Dana T, Blazina I, et al. Screening for Type 2 Diabetes Mellitus: Systematic Review to Update the 2008 U.S. Preventive Services Task Force Recommendation. 2014. Agency for Heathcare Research and Quality publication no. 13-05190-EF-1.

195 **Current recommendations are to test for abnormal blood glucose:** Siu AL. Screening for abnormal blood glucose and Type 2 diabetes mellitus: U.S. Preventive Services Task Force recommendation statement. *Ann Intern Med.* 2015; 163: 861–868.

195 **Several medications for heart disease:** Ong KL, Barter PJ, Waters DD. Cardiovascular drugs that increase the risk of new-onset diabetes. *Am Heart J.* 2014; 167: 421–428.

196 **Recommended by the Mayo Clinic:** Mayo Clinic staff. Treatment of Type 2 diabetes. Accessed at http://www.mayoclinic.org/diseases-conditions/type-2-diabetes/diagnosis-treatment/treatment/txc-20169988.

196 **Results from sixteen different studies:** Chen L, Pei J-H, Kuang J, et al. Effect of lifestyle intervention in patients with type 2 diabetes: a meta-analysis. *Metabol.* 2015; 64: 338–347.

196 **Diabetes goes hand in hand with obesity:** Golay B, Ybarra, J. Link between obesity and type 2 diabetes. *Best Pract Res Clin Endocrinol Metab.* 2005; 19: 649–663.

196 **Fat that accumulates around the abdomen:** Eckel RH, Kahn SE, Ferrannini E, et al. Obesity and Type 2 diabetes: what can be unified and what needs to be individualized? *Diabetes Care.* 2011; 34: 1424–1430.

197 **Weight loss of 5 to less than 10 percent of body weight:** Wing RR, Lang W, Wadden TA, et al. Benefits of modest weight loss in improving cardiovascular risk factors in overweight and obese individuals with Type 2 diabetes. *Diabetes Care.* 2011; 34: 1481–1486.

197 **Study conducted in Italy:** Esposito, K. Low-carbohydrate Mediterranean diet better than low-fat diet at managing diabetes. *Annals Intern Med.* 2009; 151: 306–315.

198 **Eating potatoes increased the risk of developing type 2 diabetes:** Muraki I, Rimm EB, Willet WC, et al. Potato consumption and risk of Type 2-diabetes: results from three prospective cohort studies. *Diabetes Care.* 2016; 39: 376–384.

198 **Development of diabetes with sugary soft drinks:** O'Connor L, Imamura F, Lentjes MAH, et al. Prospective associations and population impact of sweet beverage intake and type 2 diabetes, and effects of substitutions with alternative beverages. *Diabetologia.* 2015; 58: 1474–1483.

198 **130,000 diabetes deaths:** Singh GM, Micha R, Khatibzadeh S, et al. Estimated global, regional, and national disease burdens related to sugar-sweetened beverage consumption in 2010. *Circulation.* 2015; 132: 639–666.

198 **Physical activity and modest weight loss:** Colberg SR, Sigal RJ, Fernhall B, et al. Exercise and Type 2 diabetes: the American College of Sports Medicine and the American Diabetes Association joint position statement. *Diabetes Care.* 2010; 33: e147–e167.

199 **Aerobic exercise and strength training:** Sigal RJ, Kenny GP, Boulé NG, et al. Effects of aerobic training, resistance training, or both on glycemic control in type 2 diabetes: a randomized trial. *Ann Intern Med.* 2007; 147: 357–369.

200 **Metformin can cause weight loss and reduces heart attacks:** Boyle JG, McKay GA, Fisher M. Drugs for diabetes: part 1 metformin. *Br J Cardiol.* 2010; 17: 231–234.

201 **Some experts recommend against taking them at all:** Genuth S. Should sulfonylureas remain an acceptable first-line add-on to metformin therapy in patients with Type 2 diabetes? No, it's time to move on! *Diabetes Care.* 2015; 38: 170–175.

201 **People sometimes gain five to eight pounds:** Bolen S, Feldman L, Vassy J, et al. Systematic review: comparative effectiveness and safety of oral medications for type 2 diabetes mellitus. *Ann Intern Med.* 2007; 147: 386–399.

201 **This happens in up to 10 percent of people taking them:** Schopman JE, Simon AC, Hoefnagel SJ, et al. The incidence of mild and severe hypoglycaemia in patients with type 2 diabetes mellitus treated with sulfonylureas: a systematic review and meta-analysis. *Diabetes Metab Res Rev.* 2014; 30: 11–22.

202 **People taking sulfonylureas have two and a half times:** van Dalem J, Brouwers MCGJ, Krings A, et al. Risk of hypoglycemia in users of sulphonylureas compared with metformin in relation to renal function and sulphonylurea metabolite group: population based cohort study. *BMJ.* 2016; 354: i3625.

202 **More likely than other oral agents to cause hypoglycemia:** Tschöpe D, Bamlage P, Binz C, et al. Antidiabetic pharmacotherapy and anamnestic hypoglycemia in a large cohort of type 2 diabetic patients—an analysis of the DiaRegis registry. *Cardiovasc Diabetol.* 2011; 10: 66.

202 **One and a half times the number of deaths from all causes:** Morgan CL, Mukhergee J, Jenkins-Jones S, et al. Association between first-line monotherapy with sulphonylurea versus metformin and risk of all-cause mortality and cardiovascular events: a retrospective, observational study. *Diabetes Obes Metab.* 2014; 16: 957–962.

202 **Increased cancer risk:** Thakkar B, Aronis KN, Vamvini MT, et al. Metformin and sulfonylureas in relation to cancer risk in type II diabetes patients: a meta-analysis using primary data of published studies. *Metabolism.* 2013; 62: 922–934.

202 **Increased risk of heart disease:** Roumie CL, Hung AM, Greevy RA, et al. Comparative effectiveness of sulfonylurea and metformin monotherapy

on cardiovascular events in type 2 diabetes mellitus: a cohort study. *Ann Intern Med.* 2012; 157: 601–610.

203 **Two out of the top-ten-selling brand-name drugs:** Brooks, M. 100 Best-selling, Most Prescribed Branded Drugs Through June. *Medscape Medical News.* August 13, 2015. Accessed at: http://www.medscape.com /viewarticle/849457.

203 **The average price of a DPP-4 inhibitor in 2013 was $8.92 per pill:** Hua X, Carvalho N, Tew M, et al. Expenditures and prices of antihyperglycemic medications in the United States: 2002–2013. *JAMA.* 2016; 315: 1400–1402.

204 **DPP-4 inhibitors can cause severe and disabling joint pain:** FDA Drug Safety Communication: FDA warns that DPP-4 inhibitors for type 2 diabetes may cause severe joint pain. August 28, 2015. Accessed at: http:// www.fda.gov/Drugs/DrugSafety/ucm459579.htm.

204 **DPP-4 inhibitors can increase the risk for heart failure:** FDA Drug Safety Communication: Diabetes medications containing saxagliptin and alogliptin: risk of heart failure. April 5, 2016. https://www.fda.gov/Drugs/ DrugSafety/ucm486096.htm.

204 **DPP-4 inhibitors can increase the risks for acute pancreatitis:** Tucker ME. Small, but detectable, pancreatitis risk with DPP-4 inhibitors. *Medscape Medical News.* December 8, 2015. Accessed at: http://www.medscape .com/viewarticle/855583.

204 **Mouth ulcers and kidney failure:** Lowes R. Possible drug risks buried in delayed FDA 'Watch Lists.' *Medscape Medical News.* March 29, 2016. Accessed at: http://www.medscape.com/viewarticle/861078?nlid.

205 **GLP-1 agonist in the past thirty days:** Singh S, Chang H-Y, Richards TM. Glucagon-like Peptide 1 based therapies and risk of hospitalization for acute pancreatitis in Type 2 diabetes mellitus. *JAMA Intern Med.* 2013; 173: 534–539.

205 **FDA issued a communication in 2013:** FDA Drug Safety Communication: FDA investigating reports of possible increased risk of pancreatitis and pre-cancerous findings of the pancreas from incretin mimetic drugs for type 2 diabetes. March 14, 2013. Accessed at: http://www.fda.gov /Drugs/DrugSafety/ucm343187.htm#.UUH5WJ7PUnY.email.

205 **The FDA issued safety announcements about the risk of ketoacidosis:** FDA Drug Safety Communication: FDA warns that SGLT2 inhibitors for diabetes may result in a serious condition of too much acid in the

blood. Accessed at: http://www.fda.gov/Drugs/DrugSafety/ucm446845
.htm; and FDA Drug Safety Communication: SGLT2 Inhibitors: Labels
to include warnings about too much acid in the blood and serious urinary tract infections. Accessed at http://www.fda.gov/Drugs/DrugSafety
/ucm475463.htm.

206 **Safety announcement in 2015 about the possibility of bone fractures:**
FDA Drug Safety Communication. Invokana and Invokamet (canagliflozin): new information on bone fracture risk and decreased bone
mineral density. Accessed at: http://www.fda.gov/Safety/MedWatch
/SafetyInformation/SafetyAlertsforHumanMedicalProducts/ucm461876
.htm.

206 **An increased risk of leg and foot amputations with canagliflozin:** FDA
Drug Safety Communication: FDA confirms increased risk of leg and
foot amputations with the diabetes medicine canagliflozin (Invokana,
Invokamet, InvokametXR). Accessed at: https://www.fda.gov/Drugs
/DrugSafety/ucm557507.htm.

206 **SGLT2 inhibitors have recently been added to the FDA watch list:**
Lowes R. Possible drug risks buried in delayed FDA "Watch Lists." *Medscape Medical News.* March 29, 2016. Accessed at: http://www.medscape
.com/viewarticle/861078.

207 **Weight gain, swelling of extremities, and bone fractures:** Raz I. Guideline approach to therapy in patients with newly diagnosed Type 2 diabetes.
Diabetes Care. 2013; 36: Supplement 2.

207 **Increased risk of bladder cancer:** Neumann A, Weill A, Ricordeau P, et al.
Pioglitazone and risk of bladder cancer among diabetic patients in France:
a population-based cohort study. *Diabetologia.* 2012; 55: 1953–1962.

207 **An analysis of nearly 146,000 patients:** Tuccori M, Filion KB, Yin H,
et al. Pioglitazone use and risk of bladder cancer: population based cohort
study. *BMJ.* 2016; 352: i1541.

207 **Low-dose Actos is now being promoted as a preventive:** Tripathy D,
Schwenke DC, Banerji MA, et al. Diabetes incidence and glucose toler-
ance after termination of pioglitazone therapy: results from ACT NOW.
J Clin Endocrinol Metab. 2016; 101: 2056–2062.

210 **An A1c level of 7.1 to 8 is being proposed:** Allan GM, Ross D, Romney
J. Type 2 diabetes and hemoglobin A1c targets. *Can Fam Physician.* 2013
Nov; 59: 1193.

210 **Any one of five different types of drugs:** Inzucchi SE, Bergenstal RM, Buse JB, et al., American Diabetes Association (ADA), European Association for the Study of Diabetes (EASD). Management of hyperglycemia in type 2 diabetes: a patient-centered approach: position statement of the American Diabetes Association (ADA) and the European Association for the Study of Diabetes (EASD). *Diabetes Care.* 2012; 35: 1364–1379.

210 **New guidelines, issued to its medical practitioners in June 2015, recommend:** Kaiser Permanente. Type 2 Diabetes Screening and Treatment Guideline, 2015. Accessed at: https://www1.ghc.org/static/pdf/public /guidelines/diabetes2.pdf.

Chapter 10: Talking to Your Doctor

215 **People aged sixty-five or older taking five or more medications are twice as likely:** Canadian Institute for Health Information. Seniors and the health care system: what is the impact of multiple chronic conditions? 2011. Accessed at: https://secure.cihi.ca/free_products/air-chronic_disease_aib_en.pdf.

215 **One out of five prescriptions for older adults is inappropriate:** Opondo D, Eslami S, Visscher S, et al. Inappropriateness of medication prescriptions to elderly patients in the primary care setting: a systematic review. *PLoS One.* 2012; 7: e43617.

216 **Financial relationships between those producing guidelines:** Campsall P, Colizza K, Straus S, et al. Financial relationships between organizations that produce clinical practice guidelines and the biomedical industry: a cross-sectional study. *PLoS Med.* 2016; 13: e1002029.

216 **A hypothetical seventy-nine-year-old woman with five different illnesses:** Boyd CM, Darer J, Boult C, et al. Clinical practice guidelines and quality of care for older patients with multiple comorbid diseases: implications for pay for performance. *JAMA.* 2005; 294: 716–724.

Chapter 11: Making Healthy Lifestyle Changes

222 **Eighty percent of cardiovascular disease . . . could be prevented:** Yusuf S, Hawken S, Ounpuu S, et al. Effect of potentially modifiable risk factors associated with myocardial infarction in 52 countries (the INTERHEART study): case-control study. *Lancet.* 2004; 364: 937–952.

223 **Only 2.7 percent of US adults met all four requirements for a healthy lifestyle:** Loprinzi PD, Branscum A, Hanks J, et al. Healthy lifestyle

characteristics and their joint association with cardiovascular disease bio-markers in US adults. *Mayo Clin Proceed.* 2016; 91: 432–442.

223 **Eating a Mediterranean diet can reduce heart disease and deaths:** Estruch R, Ros E, Salas-Salvado J, et al. Primary prevention of cardio-vascular disease with a Mediterranean diet. *N Engl J Med* 2013; 368: 1279–1290; and Samieri C, Sun Q, Townsend MK, et al. The association between dietary patterns at midlife and health in aging: an observational study. *Ann Intern Med.* 2013; 159: 584–591.

223 **The DASH diet lowered blood pressure:** Blumenthal JA, Babyak MA, Hinderliter A, et al. Effects of the DASH diet alone and in combination with exercise and weight loss on blood pressure and cardiovascular bio-markers in men and women with high blood pressure. *Arch of Intern Med.* 2010; 170: 126.

223 **Replacing one serving of a sugary drink:** O'Connor L, Imamura F, Lentjes MAH, et al. Prospective associations and population impact of sweet beverage intake and type 2 diabetes, and effects of substitutions with alternative beverages. *Diabetologia.* 2015; 58: 1474–1483.

224 **Those who consume more refined carbohydrates and added sugars:** Gangwisch JE, Hale L, Garcia L, et al. High glycemic index diet as a risk factor for depression: analyses from the Women's Health Initiative. *Am J Clin Nutr.* 2015; 102: 454–463.

224 **People following the Mediterranean diet have less than half the inci-dence of acid reflux:** Mone I, Kraja B, Brugu A. Adherence to a predom-inantly Mediterranean diet decreases the risk of gastroesophageal reflux disease: a cross-sectional study in a South Eastern European population. *Dis Esophagus.* 2016; 29: 794–800.

225 **Ample evidence that it can reduce the risk of most chronic diseases:** Kujala UM. Evidence on the effects of exercise therapy in the treatment of chronic disease. *Br J Sports Med.* 2009; 43: 550–555.

225 **Physical activity and modest weight loss:** Colberg SR, Sigal RJ, Fern-hall B, et al. Exercise and type 2 diabetes: the American College of Sports Medicine and the American Diabetes Association joint position state-ment. *Diabetes Care.* 2010; 33: e147–e167.

226 **Exercise is as effective as medication in treating depression:** Blumen-thal JA, Babyak MA, Moore KA, et al. Effects of exercise training on older patients with major depression. *Arch Intern Med.* 1999; 159: 2349–2356.

226 **Exercise has been found to reduce the risk of falling:** Järvinen TLN, Michaëlsson K, Jokihaara J, et al. Overdiagnosis of bone fragility in the quest to prevent hip fracture. *BMJ*. 2015; 350: h2088.

226 **Physical activity three to four times a week decreases both systolic:** Eckel RH, Jakicic JM, Ard JD, et al. 2013 AHA/ACC Guideline on Lifestyle Management to Reduce Cardiovascular Risk. *Circulation*. 2014;129: S76–S99.

226 **A 64 percent increase in heart disease was found in men:** Warren TY, Barry V, Hooker SP, et al. Sedentary behaviors increase risk of cardiovascular disease mortality in men. *Med Sci Sports Exerc*. 2010; 42: 8790885.

226 **People living in walkable urban neighborhoods:** Creatore MI, Glazier RH, Moineddin R, et al. Association of neighborhood walkability with change in overweight, obesity, and diabetes. *JAMA*. 2016; 315: 2211–2220.

226 **Aerobic, strengthening, water, and tai chi exercises all improve pain:** Bennell KL, Hinman RS. A review of the clinical evidence for exercise in osteoarthritis of the hip and knee. *J Sci Med Sport*. 2011; 14: 4–9.

227 **Encouraging people to have more modest exercise goals:** P. d. S. Barreto. Global health agenda on non-communicable diseases: has WHO set a smart goal for physical activity? *BMJ*. 2015; 350: h23.

227 **Those who exercised less than 150 minutes per week:** Hupin D, Roche F, Gremeaux V, et al. Even a low-dose of moderate-to-vigorous physical activity reduces mortality by 22 percent in adults aged ≥60 years: a systematic review and meta-analysis. *Brit J Sports Med*. 2015; 49: 1262–1267.

227 **Replacing just two minutes of sitting every hour with light exercise:** Beddhu S, Wei G, Marcus RL, et al. Light-Intensity physical activities and mortality in the United States general population and CKD subpopulation. *Clin J Am Soc Nephrol*. 2015; 10: 1145–1153.

228 **The US Surgeon General's 2014 report on smoking:** US Department of Health and Human Services. The health consequences of smoking—50 years of progress: a report of the surgeon general. January 17, 2014. Accessed at: http://www.surgeongeneral.gov/library/reports/50-years-of -progress/fact-sheet.html.

228 **Long-term smokers aged sixty or above who quit smoking:** Mons U, Müezzinler A, Gellert C, et al. Impact of smoking and smoking cessation on cardiovascular events and mortality in older adults:

Meta-analysis of individual participant data from prospective cohort studies of the CHANCES consortium. *BMJ.* 2015; 350: h1551.

230 Researchers looked at the four healthy lifestyle factors: Ford ES, Bergmann MM, Kroger J, et al. Healthy living is the best revenge: Findings from the European prospective investigation into cancer and nutrition-potsdam study. *Arch Intern Med.* 2009; 169: 1355–1362.

Conclusion

240 The death rate in the United States increased in 2015: Centers for Disease Control and Prevention. Vital statistics rapid release. June 1, 2016. Accessed at: http://www.cdc.gov/nchs/products/vsrr.htm.

Acknowledgments

My biggest thank-you goes to my agent extraordinaire—Claire Gerus. Not only did she see the potential for this book in its early stages, but she also provided warm support and guidance every step of the way. Without Claire, this book would not now be in your hands. The team of editors from Skyhorse Publishing that shepherded this book also deserve to be recognized. These include Krishan Trotman, Chris Evans, Susan Randol, and finally Michael Campbell, who helped to fine-tune the finished product. Thanks also goes to Andrew Geller for his enthusiastic assistance with publicity.

I also appreciate the inspiration and feedback I received over the years from the La Paz Writer's Group, with a special shout-out to Ros Oberlin and Ulla Behn. Ros helped me to shape the earliest chapters while Ulla recognized the importance of the subject matter and encouraged me to continue writing. The Rillito River Writers Group also gave me thoughtful and timely suggestions. Several friends, including Dr. Bernardo Merizalde, Dr. Nick Nossaman, Karen Koeppler, and Patti Good reviewed selected chapters and made insightful comments. I also would like to thank the people who let me share their stories in this book. You know who you are.

Of course, I cannot close without thanking my family, especially my sweet and wonderful husband, Dean Crothers, for his constant support, encouragement, and devotion. He is my rock and most trusted adviser.

Index

About the Author

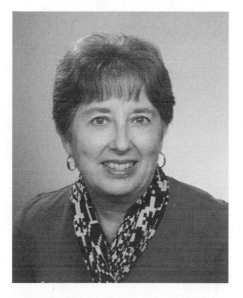

Jennifer Jacobs, MD, MPH, is a family practice physician specializing in holistic medicine. She is also clinical assistant professor in epidemiology at the University of Washington School of Public Health and Community Medicine. She has served on the advisory board of the National Institutes of Health Office of Alternative Medicine and as an advisory board member of *Natural Health* magazine. Dr. Jacobs and her husband divide their time between the Pacific Northwest and Tucson, Arizona.